how to
look great
on any budget

how to
look great
on any budget

Rosalyn Patrick

Published 2014 by Geddes & Grosset,
an imprint of The Gresham Publishing Company Ltd., Academy Park,
Building 4000, Gower Street, Glasgow, G51 1PR, Glasgow, Scotland

Copyright © 2014 The Gresham Publishing Company

Text by Rosalyn Patrick

ISBN 978 1 84205 698 1

Printed and bound in the EU

Contents

Introduction

It's your duty to be beautiful ...

We live in a looks-conscious age. Everyone is urged to look better, slimmer, smoother, more radiant, less stressed and just generally more gorgeous.

Beauty writers tell us that beauty is easy and affordable and image consultants tell us that we should make the best of ourselves. Every media outlet – from advertising to films to television to newspapers – saturates us with pictures of perfect cheekbones, glowing skin, flashing eyes and lean bodies as if, somehow, all the ordinary people (with plain brown hair and slightly pudgy thighs) have left the planet, leaving only the beautiful beings behind.

In other words, beauty is no longer something possessed by a blessed few – it is within the reach of most people, so long as they have the discipline, the right products, the right diet and the right attitude. And according to the multi-billion pound beauty industry, you now have no excuse for not looking good.

And it's certainly good to feel your best. Modern beauty products mean that boosting your looks is nothing like the chore it used to be. Few things put a spring in your step like knowing that you look well groomed are glowing with health and are dressed to impress.

An obsession

But at its most extreme, beauty can become an obsession that is impossible to satisfy. Endless, obsessive plastic surgery can result in strange and alarming results. In some cases people link beauty with happiness – they could be happy if only they looked a certain way.

Three ways for three different bank accounts

It is possible, however, to reel back some years and seriously improve your physique, without becoming obsessed or having a big bank account. This book examines the three ways (for three different types of bank account!) by which you can change the aspects of your appearance you're not happy about:—

£££ Cosmetic procedures
££ Solutions from the salon and the make-up counter
£ Changing your lifestyle and using natural remedies

£££ Cosmetic procedures

Cosmetic or plastic surgery aims to enhance the appearance, but it also includes such procedures as reconstructive surgery and skin grafting. Cosmetic surgery is plastic surgery that is only concerned with improving looks – it doesn't have a medical imperative.

The origins of plastic surgery are surprisingly ancient, and date back over 3000 years. There is evidence of early plastic surgery procedures in ancient Egyptian manuscripts, and in the writings of the Hindu doctor Susruta (*c.* 600 BC). He pioneered rhinoplasty for those disfigured by the loss of their noses, either as a punishment or in battle.

Tens of thousands of young soldiers were disfigured as a result of their wounds during the First and Second World Wars. This prompted a steep learning curve within the plastic surgery community, as surgeons worked to minimise the effects of shrapnel wounds, burns and amputations.

It has been estimated that plastic surgery made as much progress in the six years of the Second World War as it would have made in fifty years of peace. During the 1960s and 1970s the rich and famous increasingly underwent cosmetic surgery procedures.

Cosmetic surgery used to be prohibitively.expensive, but this is no longer the case, and recent surveys suggest that over half of all British women fully expect to have

13

some kind of cosmetic surgery in their lifetime. It is estimated that 11% of cosmetic procedures are now carried out on men.

Although sometimes cosmetic surgery can become an obsession, many thousands of people have had surgical procedures to enhance their breasts, lift sagging skin and exhausted-looking features, and subsequently report increased happiness and confidence.

So the industry – estimated to be worth £1 billion in the UK alone, with over 20,000 women and 2,500 men going under the knife every year – must be doing something right. The most popular treatments are breast augmentation, eyelid lifts, face and neck lifts and rhinoplasty or nose jobs.

The UK industry is well-regulated, but cosmetic surgery, like any surgery, carries risks. You should therefore ask your GP for a referral. Your GP will know who the good, local plastic surgeons are, will be in a position to inform your prospective surgeon of any relevant medical history, and will be in charge of your post-operative care.

All plastic and cosmetic surgeons must be on the General Medical Council's special register (see www. gmc-uk.org). See also the British Association of Aesthetic Plastic Surgeons (www.baaps.org.uk) and the British Association of Cosmetic Surgeons (www.b-a-c-s.co.uk).

There's a category of cosmetic procedure known as a "non-surgical" or "minimally invasive" procedure.

Introduction

£££ Cosmetic procedures

Dermal fillers, laser treatments, acid peels, cosmetic tattooing, Botox injections etc. come into this category.

Although these carry less danger to life than procedures carried out under general anaesthetic, they are certainly not without risk. These procedures are sometimes available from beauticians.

In order to minimise the risk to yourself we would advise that when choosing a practitioner you, where at all possible, only choose a doctor qualified and experienced in this area.

££ Salon and make-up counter

There is a bewildering array of beauty products and salon treatments on offer nowadays, from facial moisturisers to extraordinary creams that promise the world on a plate. Women spend an average of £3000 per year on beauty products, with male consumers and teens fast catching up.

But are these "miracle-working" products actually doing anything other than filling up your bathroom cabinet?

Opinion is as varied as the products on offer. What is clear is that while the results may be less spectacular than those of cosmetic surgery, using suitable, high quality beauty products can make a difference.

This book aims to show you how to make the most of what you've got, with a little help from your salon or the make-up and beauty counter.

£ Lifestyle and natural remedies

There are many ways of enhancing your appearance, including those that cost only effort, rather than money.

It's only relatively recently that options such as plastic surgery and intense beauty treatments have become widely available and relatively affordable, and there are many old-fashioned tonics and treatments that can be very effective. They just require a little more effort and a lot more know-how. For instance, you don't absolutely have to go to a top hairdressing salon to transform your "hair-don't" into a "hair-do". But you do need to know what suits your facial shape, what colours suit your skin tone, how to tint and streak without doing the same to your skin (or kitchen), and how to source reliable, good quality products.

You can also become your own home facialist and manicurist, without an enormous outlay. Home-made beauty can be enormous fun. You also have the freedom to experiment with all kinds of ingredients, from oatmeal to avocados and almond oil, so long as you have at least a rough idea of what you are doing with them!

Beauty, as they say, comes from within, and there's no point in investing thousands on your looks if you carry on smoking or eating a poor diet. A good lifestyle, including regular exercise and plenty of good food and rest will help you look good and slow down the ageing process.

And these kinds of changes don't need to be expensive.

Skin

Introduction

Skin is the body's largest organ, weighing in at approximately six pounds. It does a lot more than just keep the other organs from falling out. It regulates body temperature, produces sweat and sebum, stores water and fat, and facilitates our sense of touch. It also protects us from the harmful effects of ultra-violet light, and from the millions of potentially hazardous microorganisms that live in the air all around us.

Yet loving the skin you are in is easier said than done when yours flares up at the slightest provocation, is scarred, pockmarked or prematurely aged, or is paler than a shroud even after three weeks in Bermuda.

But do not despair. It is amazing what a regular dose of (fairly vigorous) exercise in the fresh air, combined with a daily one and a half litres of pure water can do for even the drabbest complexions. Add in a good diet (high in fresh fruit and vegetables and low in sugar, salt and saturated fats) good quality, regular sleep and a bright take on life and you might even discover that you don't need that face-lift after all.

On the other hand, you might feel that the only way to rejuvenate your skin or to tackle permanent blemishes is through surgery. If you decide to take this route, however, you need to take good care of your skin after surgery, or you'll probably find yourself back where you started. This includes ditching bad habits such as smoking and excessive drinking.

There is, of course, a middle way – beauty products. The beauty industry is keen to let you know all about them, even subtly hinting that certain products are as good as a face-lift. But these tend to come at a price. Don't always assume that the most expensive product is the best. Shop around, and take note of popular products – they are usually popular for a reason.

The beginning and end of good skincare, over and above the lifestyle recommendations made above, is cleansing with a good quality lotion or facial wash every night. It's best not to use soap, because this strips the skin's natural oils, leaving it sore and raw and susceptible to skin rashes and sensitivity. Men should also invest in a good quality lotion or wash that clears the pores of the dirt particles that build up during the day.

Follow this with a good quality moisturiser, ideally

with a sunscreen of at least SPF 15 for daytime, and your skin will feel and look noticeably better in a few short days. Eye-creams are a good investment for anyone over 40, as are neck creams, though both should be applied lightly and with upward strokes, to help counter the downwardly mobile effects of gravity.

Some products promise the earth and cost a fortune, so here are some good rules to bear in mind when buying a moisturiser or face cream.

First, always try before you buy. Most high-end companies offer samples, but if not, a beauty counter assistant will doubtless let you try the product, to see how you like it. This will help you to find out whether your skin will respond positively to the product, or flare up angrily at the first whiff of it.

Secondly, always use sparingly. Sloshing on skin creams can be as damaging, pore-clogging and, ironically, drying, as not using skin cream at all.

Third, seek out products containing anti-oxidants, usually billed on the packaging as vitamins A, C and E. These nutrients seem to absorb or eliminate free radicals, which damage collagen production and reduce the skin's lipid layer, where all the moisture is retained.

And finally, if the product in question is a daytime moisturiser, make sure it includes a sunscreen of at least SPF 15. Otherwise, the damaging effects of the sun, even on dull days, can cancel out all the good work your product is trying to do.

Crow's feet

Crow's feet are the fine lines that appear at the outer corners of the eyes as you age. They are caused, primarily, by the ageing process itself, when the body starts to lose some of its stocks of collagen – the all-purpose protein that gives skin its suppleness and strength. Pronounced or premature crow's feet could be the result of excessive exposure to sunlight, smoking, squinting, laughing and smiling. If they are not too deep, there is a lot you can do to mitigate your crow's feet.

£££ Cosmetic procedures

Collagen injections and dermal fillers

Non-surgical intervention, in the form of collagen injections or dermal fillers, is a boom industry. These injections claim to fill out fine lines, making the skin appear plumper and firmer. Synthetic collagen is the most popular type.

The procedure should be carried out by a certified practitioner. It begins with the application of a topical anaesthetic, followed by a series of injections, using a very fine bore needle, directly into the areas affected. These areas are then massaged, and in the following days, the filler will combine with water produced naturally by the body to produce a firmer, more youthful appearance.

The procedure can take up to an hour and you can usually leave the clinic shortly after this. The results should be apparent within one to two weeks, and can last for between three to nine months.

Allergic reactions are associated with dermal filler injections, so ensure that an allergy test is conducted beforehand, as the treatment cannot be reversed afterwards. If you are prone to cold sores, you might experience an outbreak following this treatment, unless you take anti-viral drugs as a precaution. Side-effects can also include discomfort and bruising. Serious side-effects such as prolonged redness, tissue hardness and bumps are much more rare.

Costs can vary from £200 to £1000, depending on the reputation of the clinic, the quality of the filler used, and the level of treatment you request.

Chemical peels

Chemical peels can help to reduce fine lines, but be prepared to cover up in the sun afterwards, as they leave skin thinner and more prone to sun sensitivity. A light chemical peel used to treat fine lines is quite different from a deep peel, so take good advice, preferably from a qualified dermatologist.

A light peel begins with the face being swabbed with acetone, a strong cleansing solvent. The face is then swabbed with a safe, relatively lightweight acid such as glycolic or trichloroacetic acid. Within one to two days, several layers of skin will peel off, leaving you looking noticeably rejuvenated in appearance. Several peels, applied at intervals of several weeks, may be required to make a lasting impression. A deep peel involves a much stronger acid such as phenol, and is only recommended for very deep lines or specific problems, such as scarring.

While a light peel might feel slightly nippy, a deep peel can actually be painful and a local anaesthetic might even be required. The after-effects are quite severe, with skin becoming sore, crusty and oozing until the layers peel off, leaving the face very reddened and sensitive for up to six weeks. The deeper the peel, the more severe the long-term risks. Scarring can occur, although this is rare, and changes in skin texture are also possible. About one in ten people experience an alteration in skin pigment. For this reason, chemical peels are generally recommended for very fair-skinned people only.

Chemical peels can cost from £600 to £2000 for a full course of treatment.

££ Salon and make-up counter

There is a huge array of anti-ageing potions currently on the market, but there are specific products aimed at the kind of fine lines found around the eye area.

Alpha-hydroxy acids or fruit acids

Alpha-hydroxy acids (AHAs), also known as fruit acids,

are the most prominent, and the most common form they come in is glycolic acid. As the skin ages, it becomes less efficient at sloughing off dead skin cells, causing a build-up that can leave skin looking tired and lined. AHAs cause the skin to shed these dead layers of skin through a process not unlike a chemical peel. They should be used with caution as the risks include itching, increased sensitivity to sunlight and even burns. Ideally, seek out AHAs available in products at a concentration of 10 per cent or less, and with a pH of 3.5 or less. Furthermore, avoid exposure to sunlight or wear a strong sunscreen when you are using them.

Retin-A or Tretinoin

Tretinoin, available in such products as Retin-A, is another popular, high-tech solution to fine lines. Its manufacturers claim it can actually help boost collagen production, which rejuvenates lined skin. However, use it sparingly and don't expect a result for at least a few months. It can cause itching, peeling and increased sun sensitivity, so monitor its effects as you go along – prolonged use can actually speed up the ageing process. Alternatively, use a good quality eye cream and apply sparingly, but regularly.

It's available from pharmacies, prescription only, as a cream or a gel.

Crow's feet

£ Lifestyle and natural remedies

You actually can avoid laughter lines by never laughing, but this is not necessarily recommended!

Stay out of the sun
Covering up in the sun is a great preventative measure. Always have a pair of sunglasses to hand and put them on as soon as the light is bright enough to make you squint.

Stop smoking
If you want line-free skin, then stop smoking, or don't start in the first place.

Diet
Finally, look to your diet and eat foods rich in vitamins A, C and E if you want to keep wrinkles at bay. A study of 453 Greek, Swedish and Australian people aged 70 and over was carried out in 2001 by Monash University, Melbourne, Australia. This study concluded that foods associated with younger looking skin included fresh fruit and vegetables, tea, lots of water, fish, olive oil and olives, wholegrain cereal, reduced fat milk and milk products, nuts and pulses. Foods associated with ageing skin included meat, full fat milk and dairy products such as butter and margarine, sugary foods, refined flour and, perhaps surprisingly, potatoes.

Frown lines and forehead lines

These lines start forming from a young age, particularly if you are short-sighted or short-tempered. This means that they can run deep and, unfortunately, make you look both aged and angry. As with crow's feet, there are a number of solutions to hand.

£££ Cosmetic procedures

Botox ®

The most popular non-surgical method of treating frown lines is with Botox injections. Botox – Botulinum toxin A – utilises minute, diluted quantities of the nerve toxin which causes Botulism, the paralysing, potentially fatal disease. When injected into skin, it blocks the release of acetylcholine, the chemical that triggers the contraction of muscles. Botox therefore paralyses the facial muscles whose actions, repeated over time, caused the wrinkles in the first place. Skin instantly looks smoother and rejuvenated. Over the coming months lines might fade a little, and they will be prevented from deepening.

If you have Botox treatment regularly, you could eventually find that you no longer need it, because your forehead muscles have become accustomed to non-activity.

The procedure takes around 10–15 minutes, and is conducted without anaesthetic. There is often a little bruising afterwards. Other, more serious side-effects include headache, respiratory infection, flu-like symptoms and nausea, though these are quite rare. Too much Botox can result in droopy eyelids – a problem that will correct itself as the treatment wears off. However, there is the outside possibility that your face may find another way to frown, using other muscles, thereby creating frown lines in new areas. If this is the case, then stop Botox treatments.

Positive results should be seen within days of the treatment, and should last three to four months. However, Botox only works if your wrinkles were caused by muscular activity. It has no effect on sun-damaged skin. As Botox is a prescription drug, it can only be administered by a qualified practictioner.

Botox injections cost from £175 to £300.

Dermal fillers and chemical peels
Dermal fillers, (see page 22) are another non-surgical alternative, and can be combined with Botox for longer-lasting results, or to treat very deep lines. Chemical peels are a further option (see page 23).

Forehead or brow lift
For those who want more dramatic results, and are willing and able to have surgery, then a forehead or brow lift could be an option. Brow lifts work by cutting out or partially disabling the muscles that cause the brows to contract and the forehead to rumple into horizontal lines. It is a serious operation, requiring a general anaesthetic,

and all the usual health issues must therefore be taken into consideration.

The procedure begins with an incision just under the hairline – a so-called "headphone" incision extending from ear to ear. For men experiencing baldness or hair-thinning, this incision is usually made mid-scalp, following the natural contours of the skull, to minimise visible scarring.

The skin is then lifted, underlying tissue removed and muscles released or altered. The eyebrows might also be lifted to relieve sagging. Excess skin is trimmed at the incision site, which is then closed with stitches or clips.

Alternatively, the procedure can be done using an endoscope, a tiny, pencil-like camera attached to a TV monitor. In this case, instead of a long incision three, four or five small incisions are made along the hairline, and lifted skin and eyebrows are secured subcutaneously.

As with any surgical procedure, the patient can be tired, fragile and even depressed following the operation. There will also be a degree of swelling, pain and numbness. Itching can last for up to six months. There might also be hair-thinning and scarring at the incision site.

Brow lifts cost in the region of £2700.

££ Salon and make-up counter

AHAs and Tretinoin (Retin-A)

AHAs (see page 24) and Tretinoin or Retin-A (see page 25) can also be helpful in treating frown and forehead lines.

Line fillers

Topical line fillers, which claim to plump out fine lines through boosting the production of collagen have recently reached the mass market, but no hard evidence is available as to whether they truly work. If they contain anti-oxidants, then they will at least help to combat general signs of ageing, but get youself some free samples from the beauty counter and try before you buy.

"Frownies"

Another popular treatment is "Frownies", which are patented adhesive patches applied directly to the source of the problem to inhibit frowning and moisturise intensely. They have been in circulation since 1889 and have even featured in an early Hollywood movie. They are low in cost, non-invasive and have developed a celebrity following.

£ Lifestyle and natural remedies

Relax!

The same points that apply to crow's feet also apply here. However, consciously learning to keep your forehead smooth, even in times of stress, should lead to your unconsciously maintaining a more relaxed appearance, which in turn should iron out some of those lines and halt the development of many more.

Mouth lines

Lines around the mouth are often the first, deepest and most noticeable sign of ageing on the face, and one of the greatest causes of these is smoking. The repeated puckering action by smokers causes a flurry of fine lines around the lips, while smoking itself is a major cause of premature ageing. So if you are a smoker, one of the best things you can do to reduce lines around the mouth and slow down the ageing process is to stop smoking now.

£££ Cosmetic procedures

Botox, dermal fillers, chemical peels

For lines around the mouth, you can try dermal fillers or Botox as described above, though the latter might inhibit many facial expressions while the treatment remains effective.

Chemical peels (see page 23) are a further option.

Microdermabrasion

As the skin around the mouth area is thicker than that around the delicate eye area, dermabrasion and microdermabrasion are also worth considering. Microdermabrasion is a process whereby abrasive particles – aluminium oxide or diamond crystals – are sprayed on the skin and then hoovered off, taking with them the first few layers of skin. The face should look instantly fresher and smoother, but will feel tender for a day or two.

Dermabrasion

Dermabrasion is a much harsher treatment, with the outer layers of skin literally being sanded off using a dermabrader. It is also used to treat acne scarring, and will certainly remove lines. However, it can also remove pigment, compelling you to cover up with make-up thereafter. Following dermabrasion, the skin will form a scab that heals within around ten days.

These treatments cost in the region of £80 a session.

££ Salon and make-up counter

Please refer to sections on crow's feet and frown lines on page 26.

£ Lifestyle and natural remedies

Please refer to sections on crow's feet and frown lines on page 26.

Jowls

Age, gravity and heredity can result in sagging jowls. This loose flesh overhanging a once lean jaw can be one of the most dispiriting signs of ageing, and it will only get worse as time goes on. But there are things you can do to tighten up your jowls.

£££ Cosmetic procedures

Facelift

The most radical solution to saggy jowls is a facelift, or rhytidectomy. The term "facelift" is a little misleading, because it does not refer to a full-face procedure, but to the lower third of the face, including jowls, neck and mouth. This is a pretty major operation and is usually conducted under general anaesthetic. It requires a one- to two-night stopover in hospital, plus several weeks of convalescence and follow-up appointments with your surgeon.

The procedure begins with an incision made around the front and back of the ear, following its natural contours along the hairline, so as to minimise scarring. If the surgeon uses an endoscope, then they will make several, quite tiny incisions, rather than a long, single cut. Excess fat is removed from the jowls and facial muscles are tightened to give the face a smoother, more youthful contour. This tightening is particularly important as it prevents the face from developing the "wind tunnel" effect – the notorious stretched look of early facelifts. The skin is then smoothed back, with the excess trimmed at the incision. The incision is then closed and the patient taken into recovery.

After a short stay in hospital, the patient must follow the surgeon's post-operative advice. This includes keeping the head elevated and avoiding any kind of activity that works the facial muscles too hard (for example, chewing gum) for at least several weeks. The results can be dramatic and long-lasting, providing you take care of your new face.

There are risks involved, including pain, bruising and infection. These should all be temporary. Scarring can occur but should be reasonably hidden by the hairline. There could also be loss of skin tissue near the scars or pale areas where the skin and underlying tissue were separated during the facelift procedure. Nerve damage can result in a loss of control over a certain area of the face, although this is rare.

Costs for this procedure range from £5000 to £10,000.

Threadlift: "Lunchtime facelift"

A less dramatic option with fewer associated risks is the so-called "lunchtime facelift", variously known as the "featherlift", "threadlift", "Aptos lift" and "Endo Aptos lift". This suits those aged between 30 and 50 with reasonably elastic skin and less saggy jowls.

The procedure can be carried out under local anaesthetic and involves the insertion of surgical threads beneath the skin, through incisions made at the hairline. These threads are punctuated with tiny cogs that engage with fatty tissue in the jowls. When they are pulled tight, the tissue is lifted, giving the jawline a firmer, more contoured appearance. As collagen then naturally collects at the sites of these cogs, the skin maintains its newly pushed-up configuration, making this procedure something of a guard against further premature ageing.

The risks include bumps and irregularities on the facial surface, but these usually even out in a short time. If they do not, then the threads can be removed, allowing the face to revert to its previous state.

The "lunchtime facelift" is quicker and less complicated than the regular facelift, and costs around £1500.

Liposuction

Liposuction can be performed to remove excess jowl tissue, and can be done alone, or in conjunction with a facelift. If done alone, it must be performed very carefully as even minor irregularities are very noticeable on the face. Facial liposuction should be conducted using a very small bore cannula of less than 3 mm in diameter, and should therefore be very precise.

Complications include bruising and swelling, though these should subside within a week, and improvement should be noticeable very quickly. Scarring is rare.

Costs range from about £2500 per session, for facial work.

Lipodissolve

Lipodissolve also removes excess tissue, but through a series of fat-dissolving injections rather than through a suction tube. This process is slower than liposuction, but less invasive and just as effective.

Lipodissolve can cost as little as £300 for a small area like the jowls.

Thermage and Skintyte

Treatments such as Thermage and Skintyte are even less invasive. These tighten the skin using heat-generating devices. Thermage, for example, uses a radio frequency device to deliver heat to the deep layers of the skin. This stimulates collagen, while cooling and protecting the upper layers of the skin, causing the skin to contract and tighten, and giving it a refreshed appearance. Skin should continue to improve for up to six months, when a further treatment is required to maintain improvement.

Side-effects include redness and blisters, but these should be short-lived.

A one hour treatment costs around £1500.

££ Salon and make-up counter

Don't forget your neck

When we say we take care of our skin, most of us mean that we take care of our face – stopping at the jawline. If you want to firm up a potentially sagging jawline, then your skincare needs to go all the way down to your neck.

Exfoliants

Exfoliants such as facial scrubs or grainy soaps, can help to stimulate sluggish skin by removing the outer layers of dead skin cells. Aim to give your face and jawline, a thorough but gentle scrub one or twice a week. You might have to try out a few brands before you find a product that leaves your skin clear without drying it out or causing sensitivity.

Moisturiser

A good moisturiser can work wonders too. Look for "firming" or "lifting" creams that deliver intense moisture to dry skin while also claiming to stimulate collagen production. Less is more, as with any moisturiser. Applying too much can actually make your skin drier, so use sparingly. And don't expect immediate results. It can take weeks to see an improvement.

£ Lifestyle and natural remedies

Exercise

There is a certain inevitability to saggy jowls, particularly if you have saggy-jowl genes. But you can delay the onset even without surgery and costly beauty creams. Exercise can make a difference, so try these out:

Stand up straight, with your head erect. Now slowly lift

your chin so that you are looking directly at the ceiling. Hold for 10 seconds and then lower your chin till you are looking directly at the wall. Repeat 15 times per day.

Lower your head to the left, so that your ear is facing your shoulder. Don't strain. Hold for 10 seconds, then raise your head to centre. Repeat 10 times, and then repeat for right side, again repeating 10 times.

Posture

When you are walking or sitting, try to maintain an erect head position by imagining that an invisible string is connecting the crown of your head to the ceiling. This will not only strengthen your neck muscles and help to keep the whole neck and jowl area toned, but it will also improve your deportment, giving you an instantly slimmer, more youthful demeanour.

Acne

Acne strikes most often at puberty, due to the increased production of the male hormone testosterone. This hormone, which is secreted by girls as well as boys, stimulates the production of sebum (oil). If too much sebum is produced, it can cause hair follicles, or pores, to become blocked, causing blackheads and whiteheads. Even in mild cases, the skin can feel bumpy and rough.

If the blocked pores become inflamed by bacteria, the skin becomes reddened and irritated, and nodules and cysts appear. These are unsightly and painful, and can ooze, crust or scab and leave scars. Very severe acne, called cystic acne, is rare. It can be very damaging psychologically, as well as painful and embarrassing.

Acne usually affects the face, neck and shoulders, but can also extend to the back, upper arms and even groin area.

Acne is mostly a teenage problem, but it can also affect adults (particularly pregnant women), very young children and even babies. Up to 90 per cent of us suffer from acne to some degree during some part of our lives. Boys tend to be most vulnerable, and are more likely to suffer from severe acne.

£££ Cosmetic procedures

Laser therapy

Laser therapy is the most up-to-date treatment for acne.

It is reasonably affordable and has few side-effects. At worst, it can be ineffective or is effective only as long as the treatment lasts.

There are two kinds of laser therapy recommended for acne treatment – pulsed dye laser for milder cases, and infrared for severe cases. Pulsed dye laser treatment is administered without anaesthetic, as the procedure is relatively painless. Sunglasses are usually provided to protect eyes from light damage. It is a non-ablative laser, which means that it works beneath the skin's surface to target the deeper layers of tissue and reduce the sebaceous glands that produce sebum. It also destroys bacteria and stimulates collagen production. Three sessions are usually sufficient, and there should be an immediate improvement to the appearance.

Infrared laser also works to reduce sebum production, but it can result in swelling, redness and pain, all of which are temporary It can also cause deeper pigmentation in people with darker skins, and this, unfortunately, is permanent.

A course of laser treatment costs between £1000 and £2000.

££ Salon and make-up counter

Cleansing

Most mild acne responds to a regular regime of cleansing, using a medicated facial wash to remove excess oils, dirt and dead skin cells. Look for products containing benzoyl peroxide – an anti-bacterial solution with a mild skin-peeling capacity for sloughing off the dead skin cells that exacerbate blocked pore problems.

If benzoyl peroxide reacts badly with your skin, try salicylic acid. It is obtained from white willow bark and wintergreen leaves, and it is both an antiseptic and a skin-peeling agent.

Tea-tree products can be useful too, as they are antiseptic and antibacterial. Follow twice-daily cleansing with the application of a spot cream containing sulphur, and a light, oil-free moisturiser. To reduce the appearance of acne, a gentle skin toner can wipe away oil, leaving skin looking more matte. You can also cover up with an oil-free foundation, but take care to choose one that matches your skin tone and to apply it lightly, as caking it on will only highlight your condition.

Facials

Regular facials by a beautician can also help to keep pores unblocked, but think of this as an extension of a regular cleansing routine rather than a substitute for it.

£ Lifestyle and natural remedies

Beat stress

Acne can be triggered by stress – even good stress, such as starting a new relationship. Although you can't get rid of all the potential triggers from a normal life, you can learn to cope with stress. It is beyond the scope of this book to outline in detail methods to use to counteract stress, however here are a few suggestions to research.

- Ensure you have a healthy work-life balance.
- Discuss problems when they happen – don't bottle them up.
- Try to improve your organisation skills.
- Avoid stressful people.
- Get regular exercise. Exercise is mood lifting.
- Try a fitness class such as Yoga, Tai Chi or Body Balance. Balancing is good for core fitness but also serves to concentrate the mind away from daily stresses.

See your doctor

Acne can also be caused by hormone changes due to puberty or pregnancy, or by a reaction to medication or cosmetics. See your doctor for advice if you believe your acne is linked to hormones.

Severe acne can sometimes be treated with antibiotics, which are prescribed by your GP. Visible improvement can take up to eight weeks, and courses can last as long as six months. These antibiotics can be oral or topical, but they come with the usual associated side-effects, including gastrointestinal upset. If inflammation cannot be controlled using mainstream drugs, you can be referred to a hospital skin specialist, who will prescribe stronger medication.

Also Retin-A has been found to be effective in the treatment of acne. Ask your GP if you are suitable for this treatment.

Diet

Eat a good diet rich in the skin vitamins A, C and E and drink eight glasses of water a day.

Avoid ...

If your skin is naturally sensitive, make a point of avoiding heavily perfumed products, or products that you know upset your skin. Also, avoid squeezing spots as even clean hands can and will inflame an outbreak even more and increase the likelihood of scarring, which is a beauty problem all of its own.

Blackheads

A blackhead is a pore or follicle that has become blocked with oil (sebum) and/or dead skin cells. Blackheads can occur as a result of hormone changes (for example, during puberty or pregnancy), or as a result of too much oily product (for example, sunscreen or oil-based foundation) being applied to the skin but not adequately removed at night. Initially, a blackhead is a yellow colour, which quickly oxidises to become black. Blackheads are the first stage of acne, so be careful – the wrong treatment (including no treatment) could infect and inflame your blackheads and turn them into a much more serious problem.

£££ Cosmetic procedures

Laser treatment can be used to treat both acne and severe blackheads (see page 39). Chemical peels are a further option (see page 23). However, there are salon and beauty counter remedies that might be effective.

££ Salon and make-up counter

Cleansing

Regular cleansing is the key to tackling blackheads, so invest in a good quality cleanser. Look for one that contains either benzoyl peroxide, (for its skin-peeling and antiseptic qualities) or alpha-hydroxy acid (AHA), (a skin-peeling agent, ideal for sloughing away the build-up of dead skin cells).

Prior to cleansing, steam your skin or apply a muslin cloth that has been soaked in hand-hot water for 30 seconds to open your pores and make your cleansing more effective. Afterwards, splash your face with cold water to close pores again.

Blackhead removers

Blackhead removers are a popular option for blackhead removal, and are available from any pharmacy. They should always be sterlised before use to prevent infection. Apply to the blackhead with the looped side facing down, and apply gentle pressure. If the blackhead fails to pop, do not persist, as you will almost certainly damage the skin. If you are successful, apply antiseptic cream or tea-tree oil afterwards, to ensure the area stays clear of bacteria.

Blackhead removal strips are a rather safer option and are also widely available. Do not use them too often, as they can exacerbate your condition.

Dermatologist

Even better, make an appointment with a qualified dermatologist or beautician, who can extract your blackheads painlessly and hygienically.

£ Lifestyle and natural remedies

Cleansing routine

A good cleansing routine is vital. And it needn't involve expensive branded products. Apply a solution of baking soda and water to the blackheads, rubbing it in, and then rinsing with tepid water. Or try applying warm honey and leaving it for ten minutes. Honey has a natural, skin-peeling property, and is also nourishing.

Resist the urge to squeeze them, you could cause scarring.

Hygiene

General all-round hygiene is important, such as regularly changing your pillowcase and thoroughly washing make-up sponges between uses.

Do not use make-up that is too old. Foundation should not be kept for more than 12 months.

Diet

You can also help to keep your skin clear by drinking plenty of water and eating plenty of fresh fruit and vegetables.

Whiteheads

Whiteheads are caused by dead skin cells and sebaceous matter that are trapped under the skin, a bit like blackheads. They remain a yellowish-white colour because they do not oxidise. Despite the rather benign-sounding name, they can be hard to get rid of especially as they usually occur in areas where the skin is thin and delicate, such as on the sides of the nose.

Milia are often referred to as whiteheads but milia are much more difficult to get rid of (see page 92).

££ Salon and make-up counter

Exfoliate, cleanse, moisturise

Exfoliating three to four times a week can sometimes (but not always) shift stubborn whiteheads.

If this doesn't work, book yourself in for a professional facial and commit yourself thereafter to a regimen of thorough, nightly cleansing and regular exfoliation, followed by the application of a light, oil-free moisturiser.

Piercing and squeezing whiteheads is not recommended because you can damage or infect the skin or end up with scars that take a long time to fade.

£ Lifestyle and natural remedies

Please refer to the section on blackheads on page 44.

Dry skin

Dry skin (xerosis) is a very common complaint and is characterised by a feeling of tightness (especially after washing), flakiness and a taut, slightly crepey appearance. Left untreated, it can exacerbate the formation of wrinkles and stretch marks, cause itchiness and extreme discomfort and lead to cracks, sores and even open wounds.

Dry skin is usually experienced on the legs, arms and face, and it has various causes. You might, for example, be genetically disposed to dry skin, or have underactive sebaceous glands. Winter can be a particular flashpoint for dry skin, as it is a time of low humidity, and dry air absorbs moisture from skin quite mercilessly. Summer can also be damaging, as too much exposure to sunlight can leave skin parched, even if you are wearing a sunscreen. Air travel is another cause, as is taking too many hot baths or showers, and using harsh soaps.

Dry skin is very treatable. But if conventional treatments do not work or make your skin condition worse, you might have a more severe condition such as eczema, dermatitis or psoriasis. If this is the case you should visit your GP or a professional dermatologist.

££ Salon and make-up counter

Cleanse, tone, moisturise

Regular cleansing is essential, or your skin will build up

layers of dead skin cells and wind up looking dull as well as dry. Choose a gentle, neutral pH cleanser, one that feels creamy or milky, and use morning and evening, before applying moisturiser.

If you use a toner, avoid astringent ones containing alcohol. Rose water is highly recommended.

Next, apply moisturiser in a thin layer, then allow your skin to absorb it. If it still feels taut after ten minutes, apply a second, thin layer. This will help you avoid overloading your skin and clogging pores. Choose a moisturiser that is rich and thick, and preferably oil-based. Look for one containing borage oil. This is particularly nourishing to dry skin. It is important to use a moisturiser containing suncreen (at least SPF 15) and to apply it generously when going out on cold days, so that it can serve as a barrier against harsh winds.

Hydrating mask

Hydrating masks are widely available, and are a useful way of topping up your skin's moisture levels. You can make your own by mixing a beaten egg with one teaspoonful of honey, half a teaspoonful of olive oil and a few drops of rose water. Apply and leave for ten minutes before wiping off with cotton wool or a damp cloth.

For dry skin on the body, look for body lotions designed for dry skins and massage in well. The action of massage is just as important as the product you are applying because it improves blood circulation, which in turn improves skin tone and moisture levels. You can buy skin emollients in pharmacies that you add to bathwater, or you can make your own by throwing in a handful of milk powder and a few drops of almond oil to your usual bath.

Exfoliation

Exfoliation is also important, as this sloughs away dead skin cells and keeps skin looking fresh and bright. Choose a gentle exfoliant, such as a liquid wash with a gentle skin-peeling action, and use twice a week at most. You could also try mixing coarse grain sea salt and olive oil. This will invigorate the skin while also delivering moisture to it.

£ Lifestyle and natural remedies

Drink water

It seems obvious, but drinking eight glasses of water a day will improve your skin's moisture levels. In fact, many people who think they have dry skin merely have dehydrated skin, so drinking water could cure your problem at a stroke.

Diet

Eating foods that contain plenty of water (such as raw fruit and vegetables) will also keep you hydrated, as will avoiding those foods that contain a lot of sugar and salt, such as processed foods. Fish oils are highly rated by dermatologists, so eat two to three portions of oily fish (such as salmon or mackerel) every week. If you don't like oily fish, invest in an omega supplement.

Avoid ...

Alcohol and caffeine work as diuretics and you should therefore also avoid them, or keep them to a minimum.

Having fewer baths and showers should improve dry skin, especially if they are warm rather than hot, and you stay submerged for 15 minutes or less each time. When towelling dry, pat rather than rub, and apply a thin layer of baby oil while your skin is still damp. This helps to trap a little of the moisture from your bath or shower. Leave it a few minutes, then apply your usual body lotion.

Add humidity

You can also help dry skin by installing a humidifier or by placing a dish of water on top of a radiator – this will put some humidity into the air.

Rosacea

Rosacea is also known as the "curse of the Celts" because it generally only affects white north Europeans. It is characterised by a flushed or reddened complexion and itchy, burning skin.

In time, this can develop into telangiectasia – a condition where the tiny blood vessels immediately under the skin become visible. Small white and yellow pimples can also appear and develop into pustules if left untreated. The eyes can feel dry and sore, and even become infected. In extreme cases, this can lead to infection of the cornea.

Another extreme development of rosacea is a condition called rhinophyma, where the skin on the nose becomes thickened, bumpy and purplish, giving the sufferer the appearance of a hardened drinker.

One in ten people is thought to be affected by rosacea, though women aged between 30 and 60 make up two thirds of those affected. The exact causes of rosacea are not understood, so it is impossible to prevent a first attack.

£££ Cosmetic procedures

Laser therapy

Laser therapy can be a solution for telangiectasia. Either dermatological vascular laser or intense pulsed light laser can be used because both target the layers of skin immediately underlying the epidermis. These lasers work by destroying the capillary walls, causing the body to reabsorb them. A course of laser treatment should eliminate the redness caused by visible blood vessels altogether, though follow-up treatment at a future date cannot be ruled out.

Each session, of 15–20 minutes, should cost around £300.

Dermabrasion and laser resurfacing

For rhinophyma, there are two main options – dermabrasion and laser resurfacing. Dermabrasion removes the upper layers of skin using a dermabrader, which can even out the rough skin and unsightly bumps as well as remove the discoloured skin. Dermabrasion works by wounding the skin. The wound grows new skin as it heals. The procedure requires a local anaesthetic, and sometimes a freezing (cryogenic) spray is used if the skin needs firmed up before treatment. If the abrasion is particularly deep, a general anaesthetic might even be required.

After the procedure, new skin should begin to appear within a week, but it will take from six to twelve weeks for the pinkness to fade and a more natural tone to develop.

Pain and swelling are quite common side-effects. To avoid infection, skin must be kept extremely clean, and dressings must be changed regularly to keep wounds moist. You must also avoid the sun, even after healing.

Dermabrasion costs from around £1000 upwards.

Laser resurfacing is the other main option, and it usually requires a local anaesthetic. A CO_2 laser is the one most commonly used for rhinophyma. The advantage of laser treatment is that it is very precise and works by destroying thin layers of skin. Sunglasses will probably be recommended, to protect eyes.

Again, skin will be pink and tender after the procedure, and good hygiene is essential to avoid infection.

Costs can range between £500 to £4000.

££ Salon and make-up counter

Sunscreen

Rosacea sufferers should seek gentle, hypoallergenic products and invest in a fragrance-free sunscreen for daily use with an SPF of at least 30.

Make-up

Rosacea can be very successfully disguised with clever make-up, but always use an oil-free foundation and avoid all waterproof cosmetics. The British Red Cross runs clinics on camouflage make-up and these clinics can be accessed through your local Red Cross or via a hospital skin clinic.

£ Lifestyle and natural remedies

See your GP

If pustules are the problem, then your GP will probably prescribe oral or topical antibiotics. Improvements can take two to three weeks to become apparent, and a course can typically run from six to twelve weeks.

Pustules might reappear when the antibiotics leave your system. This means that you might have to embark on a second course, or even take antibiotics on a semi-permanent basis.

An alternative to antibiotics is azelaic acid, which can be applied topically. However, this can make the skin very dry and flaky, or sting and itch.

Avoid ...

Though the root causes are unknown, rosacea seems to be triggered by certain kinds of food or drink or atmospheric conditions. Hot and cold food, alcohol (particularly red wine), spicy food and caffeine are common triggers. The National Rosacea Society recommends that you keep a food diary to pinpoint what your trigger might be, so that you can then eliminate it from your diet.

Extreme heat or cold (and alternating between the two) can be a trigger, as can windburn and sun exposure. It's therefore a good idea to avoid such extremes.

Men often find that switching from a razor blade to an electric shaver can be helpful.

Steroid creams are another possible trigger, and should be avoided. If you feel that a course of medication has caused or exacerbated your rosacea, speak to your GP, who can prescribe an alternative.

Cleansers containing alcohol or acetone should also be avoided, as should harsh exfoliants and heavily fragranced products.

Thread veins

Thread veins – also known as spider or broken veins – are the tiny red veins that sometimes appear on cheeks, nose, legs and body. "Broken veins" is actually a misnomer The veins are not broken at all – rather, the capillary walls have become weak and the blood is therefore visible through them. The veins are even more visible on thinning, ageing skin.

The causes are various and include genetic predisposition, too much exposure to the sun, pregnancy, a boost of the female hormone oestrogen through HRT or the contraceptive pill, or the use of steroid creams. Middle-aged women are most vulnerable. As with rosacea, certain foods and drinks seem to act as a trigger, so it is often worth cutting down on alcohol, caffeine and spicy foods, or keeping a food diary to identify the cause. In most cases, effective make-up will cover up thread veins, but treatments are available for those that defy the concealer stick.

£££ Cosmetic procedures

There are two main treatments for thread veins – laser therapy and microsclerotherapy.

Microsclerotherapy
Microsclerotherapy is recommended for treating thread veins on the legs.

Skin

Thread veins

The procedure (which can take from 30 minutes to one hour) works through the injection of an irritant solution into the problem veins. This then causes them to collapse. The body treats these collapsed veins as waste tissue and reabsorbs it. It is important that the practitioner injects accurately, as solution injected into skin by mistake can cause irritation and discolouration.

Normal activities such as driving a car are possible immediately. Support stockings are recommended for up to a week after treatment.

Swelling and freckle-like marks at the injection sites, are common side-effects, but these should both be short-lived. Sometimes treated veins can turn black, though these should start to fade within three weeks, and vanish completely by three months.

You might need as many as five treatments to get rid of thread veins. You should also note that although the treatment permanently destroys existing veins, it won't prevent you from developing new thread veins elsewhere, especially if you are predisposed to them.

Costs range from £150–£250 per session.

Laser treatment

Laser treatment destroys the veins under the skin using a pulse of light, and is suitable for removing thread veins on the face. Side-effects can include bruising, textural changes to the skin and little white scars

A third treatment is Photoderm or hi-intensity light

treatment, where a flash of pulsed light is directed at a section of the face (roughly 2 mm by 0.5mm) causing the veins to coagulate and disappear. It is a reasonably painless procedure, similar to being flicked in the face. Side-effects can include a temporary reddening and swelling.

Costs start at £150 per session.

££ Salon and make-up counter

Concealer

When it comes to thread veins, concealer is your best friend, so choose a good quality product, and one that blends in with your skin tone. Apply by dabbing or patting, rather than trying to rub it in, and use prior to applying foundation.

Fake tan

Fake tanning is another good way to disguise thread veins. (Don't confuse this with sunbed tanning, which could exacerbate your condition.) Take care to exfoliate skin carefully before applying fake tan to avoid a streaky effect. Better still, pay a professional beautician to do it for you.

Horse chestnut

Consider investing in a skin cream containing horse chestnut extract, which has had very positive results in the treatment of both thread and varicose veins. Horse chestnut is a natural capillary strengthener, but long term use is essential – you won't get immediate results.

£ Lifestyle and natural remedies

Avoid

If thread veins on legs are a problem, try to avoid standing still for prolonged periods and aim to sit with your legs elevated for at least 20 minutes a day.

Massage

Massaging the face and legs can also help, as it keeps the blood flowing and prevents the veins from becoming weak.

Scarring

The formation of scar tissue following injury or inflammation is an essential part of the healing process. However, when scars are visible, uncomfortable, unsightly or when they hinder movement, then you might want to give nature a helping hand. Most scars fade with time to become virtually invisible. But some don't. Sometimes, the wound "overheals" through the overproduction of collagen at the site and this causes raised, angry-looking scars.

Hypertrophic scars are caused by this process, but stay within the boundaries of the original wound site because they stop producing collagen once the wound has healed. They usually fade with time, though certain procedures and treatments can speed the process along, and make the fading more pronounced.

Keloids are also the result of too much collagen, though in this case they keep on producing collagen long after the wound has healed, and eventually invade the surrounding skin area. They are raised, sometimes claw-like scars that are often pink or purple, and can also be painful and itchy. They mostly occur on the back, chest and arms, though rarely the face. They can cause considerable distress and are often troublesome to treat.

Indents or flat scars caused by acne are relatively minor problems, though all things are relative and they can be very distressing. This kind of scarring is treatable with surgery and through non-invasive methods. It is important to note that general good health and good wound care will go a long way to preventing any scarring in the first place. Of course, some people scar more easily than others, and this can be down to age, genetics, skin colour, and the nature of the wound. However, if you keep the area clean, consult a GP about whether it should be sutured (this keeps the wound closed and minimal), and keep it moist (dry wounds scar more than wet ones), you will keep damage to a minimum. Sunblock is another prerequisite, as UV light interferes with the healing process and can cause increased pigmentation.

£££ Cosmetic procedures

Revision surgery

Having surgery on an existing scar can make it much worse, so approach with caution. Revision surgery is sometimes recommended as a treatment for raised scarring, such as keloids, and is a process where the scar is surgically removed, often under general anaesthetic, then stitched up. This will hopefully achieve a flatter, smoother scar. However, there is always the possibility that the body will reproduce the process that caused the original scar, and a bigger scar might result.

Cryotherapy

Cryotherapy uses liquid nitrogen to freeze off keloids,

with the nitrogen blasted at the site for 15 to 30 second periods, causing the cells to die. Though quite a simple and safe procedure, cryotherapy can be painful and can result in increased pigmentation of the skin.

Costs begin at £100, or even less.

Cortisone injections

Another course of action is to anticipate and interrupt the formation of raised scars, particularly if you have already developed one keloid in your life. Micro-injections of cortisone, for example, can interrupt the process of collagen overproduction and ensure minimal scarring. This procedure is painless and safe, as very little cortisone reaches the bloodstream. However, it can make the site more red and sensitive by stimulating the production of red blood cells.

Dermabrasion

Dermabrasion (see pages 32 and 53) can also be effective on raised scar tissue. For indents, collagen injections will raise scars to the natural skin level, but the effects are short-lived – about four months.

Dermabrasion costs around £150 per injection.

Laser treatment

Laser treatment that is targeted at underlying skin tissue can promote collagen production, but can take up to six treatments to be effective. This can be an effective and long-lasting solution to indented scars if it is followed up by microdermabrasion (see page 31). It is, however, quite a painful procedure and can require up to two weeks' recovery time.

The full treatment costs around £300.

££ Salon and make-up counter

Silicone gels

Creams and gels can help to minimise scarring and promote fading. Silicone is the key ingredient to look out for, as it is instrumental in helping scars to heal. Silicone gels are effective, as are silicone sheets, which can be worn for prolonged periods of time and not only aid fading, but also flatten scars out over time. Two to four months of silicone application can make a substantial difference.

Pressure dressings

Pressure dressings also help to flatten scars and are generally used for large-area damage, such as burns. They might have to be worn for up to a year, and can be uncomfortable in hot weather, but are effective and risk-free.

Mederma™ *gel*

Mederma gel, a patented product, contains onion extract, and can help to reduce scar tissue formation.

Bio Oil™

Bio Oil™ is formulated to help fade scars and stretch marks. It is claimed it can even improve the appearance of old scars, and clinical trials have shown it to be effective in this way for around 65 per cent of users. It is especially effective in improving uneven skin tone. The oil is made from PurCellin Oil™, vitamin A and vitamin E; and calendula, lavender, rosemary and chamomile esssential oils.

Skin concealers

Skin concealers are also very useful tools, though dry ones are more likely to adhere than oily ones. For large areas, choose a corrective foundation, ensuring that it matches your skin tone and adheres to the scar tissue effectively.

£ Lifestyle and natural remedies

See your GP

Hydroquinone-based fading creams (available from your doctor on prescription only) can also reduce the appearance of scars, though side-effects include redness, itching and increased sun sensitivity.

Massage

As mentioned, good health and wound care are essential. Massage will help to break down the collagen in raised scars, but this should be done gently and regularly and only once the scar tissue has formed, otherwise you run the risk of stretching the wound further.

Salt water

Salt water has long been recommended as a natural promoter of skin healing, and can do little harm so long as you do not expose your skin to too much sunlight while you are in it.

Vitamin E

Vitamin E is often quoted as a great all-round skin ingredient, so if you can't apply it, eat it, as this will help your skin heal too.

Licorice extract

Licorice extract is another useful ingredient, as it is a natural skin lightener.

Sun damage

Once upon a time, the sun was considered a major beauty treatment in itself. The "Beautiful People" always sported a serious Riveria suntan. But we have learnt a great deal about the damaging effects of UV exposure since the 1970s. Indeed, all the signs that we associate with ageing – wrinkles, leathery and sagging skin – might in fact be due solely to sun damage, or photoageing.

Sun damage does not just occur in those who sunburn regularly, or are constantly baking themselves under sunbeds, nor does it become fully apparent for many years. The most common problems associated with too much sunlight are lined and sagging skin, freckling, a yellow tint, and leatheriness. Pores may also become enlarged.

More serious is solar keratosis, also known as actinic keratosis, which alters the size, shape and structure of skin cells, resulting in crusty lesions up to 1 inch in diameter. These may be light or dark brown, pink, red or simply your own skin colour, in which case they are generally first detectable by touch, being raised, with a rough texture and possibly a crust on top. They may feel tingly and itchy, and occur most often on the face, arms, hands and shoulders – the areas most likely to be exposed over a long period of time to the sun.

If you suspect solar keratosis, you should always consult your GP, as one in ten cases can become cancerous and the earlier the detection, the better the prognosis.

Though it can look alarming, and feel uncomfortable, solar keratosis often just goes away all by itself, over the course of one or two years, so long as you keep the affected skin out of the sun. If it changes size or shape, or becomes tender within that time, it is important that you seek medical advice. The treatment options for sun damaged skin are improving all the time, but prevention is far better than cure and it cannot be overstated how important proper sunscreen is, from infancy onwards.

£££ Cosmetic procedures

Solar keratosis can be treated in a number of different ways.

Cryotherapy

Cryotherapy (as described on page 61) will freeze off lesions, and the site will then blister and scab, ultimately resulting in a (hopefully) scar-free skin. Lesions can also be cut out surgically, and the wound stitched up, but this is not often recommended unless there is a medical imperative. Cautery is another option, where the lesion is scooped out using a surgical spoon, and the site is then cauterised. This is simpler than surgery, but will leave small, indented scars.

Costs start from £50.

Topical applications

Topical applications are less invasive, but they are not

without complications. Your GP might prescribe a gel or cream containing the anti-inflammatory drug Diclofenac, which is usually only effective only after three months' use. The drug flourouracil kills abnormal cells, allowing new ones to grow in their stead, but although the full treatment only lasts for four weeks, it often causes blistering and inflammation.

Laser brasion

For more general sun damage, laser brasion is a popular choice, where an Erbium Yag laser removes the skin, literally vaporising it, to allow new, healthy skin to grow in its place. This process can be painful and requires a prolonged recovery time, due to redness of the skin and sensitivity. It can also result in damage to skin pigment.

Non-ablative laser surgery

Non-ablative laser surgery is less risky and comes with fewer side-effects, because it targets underlying tissue to stimulate collagen, thereby helping the skin to renew itself.

Laser treatments start at about £1000 per session, though packages are sometimes available for a series of sessions.

££ Salon and make-up counter

AHAs

Products containing alpha-hydroxy acids (AHAs) or

glycolic acid, which have skin-peeling properties, can be used to rejuvenate skin that is prematurely aged by the sun, resulting in a smoother, more even complexion. But cover up well afterwards, as these products can make skin extremely sun sensitive (see also page 24).

Vitamin C

Vitamin C is also a useful ingredient in moisturisers and other skin products because it boosts the skin's ability to renew itself and turn over dead cells.

Tretinoin or Retin-A

Tretinoin – available on prescription only – can thicken skin thinned by UV exposure. It can also reduce pigmentation by inhibiting the skin's melanin production. But it only works over a long period of time, so be persistent.

Tazarotene

Tazarotene (generally recommended for psoriasis) is another effective agent against sun damage.

Astringent toner

To help tighten pores, invest in a good quality astringent toner, and use after cleansing and before moisturising.

Sunblock

Finally, get a good sunblock and use every single day, no matter what the weather.

£ Lifestyle and natural remedies

Avoid ...

If you want to avoid or minimize sun damage to skin, you should avoid direct sunlight. Cover up what you can with clothes and cover up what you can't with a sunscreen of at least 15 SPF. Try to avoid the sun between 11 am and 3 pm, and stick to shady areas.

Diet

We've said it before, but we'll say it again. A good diet, with plenty of fresh fruit and vegetables and water, will help your skin enormously, as will regular moisturising.

Natural preparations

To tighten pores, splash your face morning and night with cold water, or use a solution of cucumber, rosewater and a few drops of chilled witch hazel over skin after cleansing.

Egg whites make a good pore tightening mask. Apply over the skin and allow to dry.

An almond paste mask – made by pulverising skinless almonds into a powder and adding rose water – helps to improve skin elasticity.

Sleep

Plenty of regular sleep will also boost your skin's ability to grow new, healthy cells.

Stretch marks

Stretch marks, as the name suggests, are caused by over-stretching of the skin, to the extent that it loses its ability to snap back into shape. This is because the underlying tissue becomes weakened, causing layers of skin to separate. Stretch marks start out as red, brown or purple grooves or indents that gradually fade to a silvery-white as they heal. This healing process concludes with a burst of collagen production (or over-production) that results in raised scar tissue.

Stretch marks are most common on the hips, breasts, buttocks, thighs, abdomen and arms. People with dry skin seem to be more prone than those with normal or oily skin. Stretch marks can appear as a result of pregnancy, puberty, sudden weight gain or loss – any event that entails sudden growth. It might simply be the physical act of stretching that causes the marks, or the hormonal reaction to the sudden growth.

Other causes include the over-use of steroids and Cushing's Syndrome. Age, body mass index, genes and skin colour all play a part in determining how severe stretch marks will be, but there is a range of treatments on offer to mitigate their development and reduce their appearance.

£££ Cosmetic procedures

Surgery is not recommended for the treatment of stretch

marks, as this often means simply replacing pale, fading scars with bright, new ones.

Laser treatment

Laser treatment is the preferred treatment, though it is only effective on new stretch marks, not faded ones. Fractional laser therapy involves a fine laser creating a series of microscopic wounds in the skin, leaving a channel of healthy skin in between. This healthy skin helps the wounds to heal over with new, healthy skin cells. It can be an unpleasant, rather than painful treatment and requires several sessions.

Pulsed Dye laser targets the underlying tissue, making the blood vessels seal up, thereby reducing the redness of new stretch marks and speeding the fading process. Note that the marks would fade anyway, though over a longer period. Again, several sessions are required, with improvements often discernible for up to six months.

Costs start at around £1000 per session, with discounts sometimes available for a series of sessions.

Endermologie

Endermologie is a French, non-invasive treatment, generally used to treat cellulite, which has had some success with stretch marks. The skin is massaged with rollers, which helps to redistribute fatty tissue. The rollers also have a suctioning action, which is claimed to improve blood circulation by up to 200 per cent. The procedure works by stretching and strengthening connective tissue, resulting in smoother skin It can be a very invigorating treatment and patients are often required to wear a body stocking before the rollers are applied. A series of sessions are required, with each lasting around 30–45 minutes.

Sessions cost around £50.

Microdermabrasion

Microdermabrasion (see page 31) can help to give skin a smoother appearance, and can produce results in the treatment of stretch marks, especially if used in combination with products such as Retin-A or Tretinoin (see below).

££ Salon and make-up counter

Moisturise

The key word with regard to stretch marks is prevention, so if you are vulnerable, start moisturising now – up to three times a day. Look out for vitamins A and C (the skin-nourishing vitamins), wheatgerm, cocoa butter (a useful ingredient in the treatment of scars), grapeseed oil and jojoba in your products.

Skin creams will certainly help to relieve the itchiness of stretched skin and will help to reduce the severity of stretch marks, if not actually prevent them.

Tretinoin (Retin-A)

Tretinoin, commonly known as Retin-A (available only on prescription) is sometimes effective, but only on new stretch marks. It should not be used during pregnancy or while breastfeeding, as it can potentially harm your baby. Tretinoin thins the skin, boosting new growth.

AHAs

Alpha-hydroxy acids can be effective too, as they essentially burn off old skin cells, stimulating the production of new ones (see page 24).

£ Lifestyle and natural remedies

Massage

Massaging your own stretch marks works like a low-key Endermologie session (see page 72), but must be done regularly if noticeable results are to be achieved. Many skin experts insist that the massage is more important than the cream you are rubbing in, so don't be discouraged if you can only afford budget moisturisers.

Diet

Diet is also important. Maintain a healthy weight, drink plenty of water, and eat foods containing vitamins A and C and silica, which can assist the production of collagen.

Excess skin

Congratulations! You've just lost five stone!

And commiserations! Your skin hasn't realised it yet.

A sting in the tail of a major weight loss campaign can be the folds of loose, excess skin left behind. Not only is excess skin unsightly and often uncomfortable – it can even be the source of minor but irritating health problems, because fungus can develop between those folds, causing itchiness and broken skin.

A heavy pregnancy can also leave you with excess skin, and this can be exacerbated by having a Caesarean section, as the muscular wall of the abdomen has been severed, making it much harder to tighten up and become firm. In time – sometimes up to two years – loose skin does generally become firmer, but only if you maintain a steady weight and exercise regularly. Age and skin type all play a part too.

£££ Cosmetic procedures

People often think that surgery is the best solution for excess skin. You are, however, usually advised to exhaust all the other possibilities first, and you need to have maintained your ideal weight for at least two years before this is an option. Women who are planning further pregnancies are advised to hold off too, as the effects of surgical procedures will only be undone.

Abdominoplasty or tummy tuck

For the removal of excess skin, one of the most popular procedures is the abdominoplasty, or tummy tuck. This is a major operation, conducted under general anaesthetic, and can take anything between two to four hours.

The surgeon begins by making an incision along the bikini line, just above the pubis, usually extending from hip to hip. The naval will then be cut away and put to one side, to be replaced at the end of the operation.

A flap of abdominal skin is cut and pulled back, so that the surgeon can draw up the vertical abdominal muscles till they are taut, then suture them into position. (Any excess fat can also be removed at this point by using liposuction, which suctions away the fatty tissue.)

The flap is then stretched down to the incision line, excess skin is trimmed away (which also gets rid of any stretch marks), and the wound is stitched. The naval will then be replaced at the appropriate position. Drains will probably be inserted to draw off excess fluid, and these are removed after a few days. The result should be a firmer, smoother stomach and reduced waist. This can last for a decade, if you take good care of your body.

A tummy tuck is the same as any other major operation. Many tummy tuck patients require a two or three night stay in hospital, though getting up and walking around is advisable as soon after the operation as possible, to avoid blood clots. Post-operative pain and discomfort are almost inevitable, and are treated appropriately and should subside within a few days. You can return to work within two to four weeks, though you have to wait longer before you can resume vigorous exercise, and it will take from nine months to a year before the (discreet) scarring will start to fade.

This procedure will cost up to £8000.

Endoscopic tummy tuck

A less invasive procedure is the endoscopic tummy tuck. Here, a series of small incisions are made instead of one long one, and a camera device is inserted to allow the surgeon to draw up the vertical muscles and tighten them, before sealing off the incisions.

Lower body lift

A more serious take on the tummy tuck is the lower body lift, which includes a lifting of the abdominal area, as described above, and a thigh and buttock lift. A thigh lift requires incisions to be made in the upper, inner or outer thigh, followed by removal of excess fatty tissue and stretching of the thigh and buttock skin upwards towards the incision. Excess skin is then trimmed and the wound stitched. This operation can take up to six or seven hours, and is not for the faint-hearted. However, if successful, the transformation can be remarkable.

As you would expect, healing takes longer than with an abdominoplasty, due to the extra number of incisions and the longer time spent in surgery. Rest, gentle movement and excellent consultant after-care are required. Be prepared for pain, discomfort and numbness in some areas, as nerves seek to recover. There will probably also be some scarring, which should eventually fade.

This procedure can cost up to £15,000.

££ Salon and make-up counter

If you cannot stomach surgery, then be prepared for a long haul. That said, the results can be dramatic, if you stick at it.

Exfoliation
Daily exfoliation is highly recommended, as this will slough off dead cells and prompt the skin to repair itself and tighten up.

Skin firming creams
Skin firming creams are also useful, but require persistence. Ingredients to look for include hyaluronic acid, (which claims to boost the production of collagen fibres, lending skin increased elasticity) and fibrillin (a protein associated with the production of collagen). Look out too for antioxidants, which reduce the damaging action of free radicals, and often come in the form of grapeseed oil and vitamins A, C and E.

£ Lifestyle and natural remedies

Exercise

Maintaining a steady weight is key, as is regular exercise, especially if it is targeted at the problem areas. If you can afford it, employ the services of a personal trainer, at least to start you off. Such a professional can see where the problems lie and draw up an exercise regime tailor-made for you.

Freckles and liver spots

Freckles are tiny, tan-coloured spots that appear following exposure to the sun. They are most common in fair and red-haired people with pale skin and blue eyes. They are, however, not unavoidable, or "natural". A young child covered in freckles has simply had more exposure to UV rays than their skin can cope with. Freckles are caused by an over-production of melanin, the skin's pigmentation agent, which is produced when the skin needs protection from the sun.

Liver spots are the old-age version of freckles, and generally appear after the age of 55. They are also known as senile lentignes, or old age spots, and most frequently appear on the face and hands, where the skin is thinnest and most likely to be exposed to the sun. Liver spots have nothing to do with the liver. They are usually tan-coloured, like freckles, but can sometimes be a reddish-brown, the colour of liver. They range from freckle-sized to up to an inch or so in diameter. They are rarely cancerous, but liver spots have clearly defined edges, so any change in shape, size or colour should be investigated by your GP, especially if you have a family history of malignant melanoma. The best treatment is of course prevention, so if you are inclined to freckle and are already showing signs of liver spot development cover up, use a sunblock and whenever possible avoid the sun between the peak hours of 11am and 3pm.

£££ Cosmetic procedures

Microdermabrasion

For freckles, a skin-resurfacing treatment such as microdermabrasion can produce significant improvements, though several sessions are probably necessary.

Costs begin at £50 per session.

Chemical skin peels

Chemical skin peels are also a good option, though it is vital to cover up in the sun afterwards, as skin will become particularly photo-sensitive. (See pages 23–24.)

Costs can range from £60 to £1500, if damage is extensive.

Cryotherapy

For liver spots, cryotherapy (where liquid nitrogen is used to freeze the problem area) is effective, but can be uncomfortable or even painful, and runs the risk of leaving you with permanent white scars.

Prices start at £50.

Laser treatment

Laser treatment is less painful, less invasive and less likely to scar.

Costs begin at £500.

££ Salon and make-up counter

There are several creams and gels that might be effective. However, if any of these products causes itchiness or redness, discontinue use immediately as it is clearly too powerful for your particular skin. Ask your GP for advice.

Skin-bleaching or spot-fading creams

Skin-bleaching or spot-fading creams are very effective at reducing the appearance of both freckles and liver spots. Hydroquinone is the key ingredient to look for. It works by shutting down the production of melanin in problem areas, causing spots to fade over time. Hydroquinone is recommended for fair skins only, while kojic acid, a Japanese discovery, is suitable for all skin types and is a gentle, plant-derived substance. It too works by inhibiting melanin production, causing gradual fading of pigmentation.

AHAs

Alpha-hydroxy acids or AHAs (in gel form) are a further option, producing significant lightening after several weeks of daily (or rather, nightly) application. (See page 24.)

Retin-A (Tretinoin)

Prescription-only Retin-A, or Tretinoin, lightens large spots and reduces small ones until they have almost disappeared. (See page 25.)

Make-up

If all else fails, you can cover up with a good foundation, though take advice from a make-up expert and find a tone that matches your own, to avoid a mask-like appearance. Foundations are also available for use on the body, including the hands.

£ Lifestyle and natural remedies

Avoid the sun

The best advice is to avoid sunlight. Invest in a good sunblock, a hat and long sleeves to see you through the summer, and remember to also cover up in winter, when although the weather is cold the sun can still be strong.

Lemon juice

The application of lemon juice to freckles and liver spots can result in significant fading. Slices of other acidic fruits are also effective.

Cellulite

Cellulite is the dimpled, "orange peel" skin that appears on the thighs, hips and stomach – predominantly of women – anytime after puberty. Cellulite is experienced by around 90 per cent of all women (and some men too) many of whom are otherwise toned, slim and healthy. It occurs in the subcutaneous layer of skin where fibrous connective tissue, called septa, holds fat cells in place. These fat cells are essential for keeping the body warm and bolstering the structure of the skin itself. But if the fat cells become slightly displaced, forming clusters, they appear as bulges under the outer layer of skin. Obese people are much more prone to cellulite because their lower layers of fat push the subcutaneous layers outwards.

We have no clear idea what causes cellulite. What we do know is that it is more common as you age, when the outer layer of skin becomes thinner and less effective at smoothing over bumps. We also know that men are less susceptible, partly because they naturally have less body fat, produce more collagen (which makes their skin more elastic) and have a different septa structure. Sluggish circulation, poor lymphatic drainage, fluid retention, female hormones, obesity and smoking are all cited as major aggravators of the condition and, as you might expect there are many "cures" available to try – some might work and some simply won't work.

£££ Cosmetic procedures

Liposuction

It's not clear how effective liposuction is at removing cellulite. It's a reasonably simple procedure, involving the insertion of a very thin, hollow tube, called a cannula, into tiny incisions in the skin. Excess fat is then carefully suctioned out to avoid nerve and tissue damage. The incisions are then sutured.

The procedure can take several hours, and can leave you very sore and swollen. (The swelling can remain for several weeks.) You are advised to wear a girdle throughout the recovery period to help the skin resume a natural shape and keep swelling to a minimum.

Side-effects can be life-threatening but are extremely rare. These include small clots of loosened fat and blood clots, which can be fatal if they reach the lungs, and the loss of too much fluid, which can also be very dangerous. Though liposuction can make cellulite disappear, it can also damage the lymphatic system and make the area even more prone to the development of cellulite in the future.

Liposuction can cost from £5000 to around £8000.

Fat injections

Another option is fat injections, where fat is harvested from elsewhere on the body. These injections work by filling out the bumpy skin, giving it a smoother contour. However, this effect is only temporary as the fat is gradually reabsorbed by the body, usually within six months.

Fat injections cost from £150 upwards.

Lower body lift

If you are having a lower body lift to lift your tummy, thighs and bottom then this will automatically get rid of your cellulite (see page 77). This is an extreme operation not recommended just for cellulite removal!

Mesotherapy

Mesotherapy is a procedure where homeopathic medicine, minerals and vitamins are injected into the subcutaneous layer, where they are said to help to break down cellulite formation by stimulating circulation and lymphatic drainage. Injections take around ten minutes each, and a series is recommended, depending on the extent of the problem. Improvement is temporary.

Costs range from £150 to £300, per body part, per treatment.

Endermologie

Endermologie (see page 72) is another option, but again with short-term results. Accent Radio Frequency is a reasonably comfortable and non-invasive treatment, and works by deep-heating the subcutaneous layer, while keeping the outer one cool. It claims to stimulate the formation of collagen, boost blood circulation, and shrink fat cells.

Manual Lymphatic Drainage massage

Manual Lymphatic Drainage (MLD) massage encourages the lymphatic system to work better and relieves fluid retention. It does this through a light, soothing massage. Improvement is temporary. Costs range from £50 to £150.

££ Salon and make-up counter

Tretinoin (Retin-A)

Tretinoin or Retin-A, appears to be the only product that even scientists agree reduces cellulite, but it is prescription-only. It works by thickening the outer layer of skin, reducing the appearance of cellulite. Its over-the-counter version, Retinol, can be effective, but only over a long period of time.

Demethylaminoethanol

Other cellulite-busting favourites include demethyl-aminoethanol or DMAE. This is an antioxidant made from fish, combined with amino acids, and is claimed to have a significant skin-tightening effect.

Caffeine

Caffeine is now used in the fight against orange peel skin, and works by flushing the water out of fat cells, making them smaller and therefore less noticeable. But it is only a very quick fix, and probably not that good for you in the long run, as dehydration can degrade the appearance of skin.

£ Lifestyle and natural remedies

Diet

A good diet is top of the list for tackling cellulite. You should reduce processed and salty foods, dairy products and tea, coffee and alcohol to a minimum, while increasing your intake of fresh fruit, vegetables and water. This way, you'll encourage good digestion and avoid fluid retention.

Exercise

Exercise is also important – particularly if the exercise is targeted at problem areas. Tight clothing, especially underwear with tight elastic, can be a contributing factor, so opt for breathable fabrics that don't squeeze your skin and inhibit good circulation.

Relax

Reducing stress may also make a big difference, so taking time to relax, get into a good sleep pattern and find a good place to be emotionally should have knock-on benefits for your appearance, including cellulite.

Body brushing

Finally, body-brushing with a dedicated, soft body brush can have a great impact on dimpled skin. Use daily before your shower or bath using long, soft strokes (always towards the heart) and moisturise well afterwards.

Skin tags

Skin tags are also known as acrochordons and cutaneous papilloma. They are small tumours that appear like nodules of skin hanging from a stalk. They are usually tiny and flesh-coloured, but can also be brown and grow to the size of a grape. They usually occur in areas where skin rubs against skin (for example in the groin area, the armpits, neck and eyelids) and where tight clothing rubs against skin (for example, where underwired bras rub against the skin under the breasts).

Skin tags are generally age-related. They usually occur in people over 30, but they can also appear as a result of pregnancy hormones or type 2 diabetes. They range from barely visible to extremely unsightly, and often snag on clothing and jewellery, becoming inflamed and even bleeding. However, they are almost never cancerous and there is rarely a medical imperative for removal. Removal can be a very simple matter but it is considered a cosmetic procedure so is not available on the NHS.

£££ Cosmetic procedures

Burning or freezing
Skin tags can be burnt off using electrolysis, or frozen off using liquid nitrogen. These are quick and easy methods, but can cause discolouration and may, in fact, not always work.

Excision

Skin tags can also be excised using a scalpel, which can lead to minor bleeding. Usually, all three methods can be conducted without anaesthesia. However, a topical anaesthesia will probably be applied when tackling larger growths. It will probably cost from £50 per small area of treatment. Ask a doctor for advice or see a skin specialist.

££ Salon and make-up counter

Dermisil

Ask your GP's advice first, to be sure that what you are dealing with really are skin tags and not any other kind of skin growth. If they are true skin tags and not moles, there are a number of herbal remedies on the market that are designed to make skin tags dry up and flake off. Dermisil is one such product, and is based on plant extracts. Reviews are mixed.

Nail polish

Clear nail polish is a cheaper method, and should be applied daily to the skin tag until it disappears. It requires a little patience, but the acid in the polish should eventually be effective.

£ Lifestyle and natural remedies

As obese people have more folds of skin than slim ones,

they are also more likely to develop more skin tags. If you watch your weight, you may also help to prevent skin tags.

If skin tags are already present, there are a number of DIY remedies, but before trying them you must ask a doctor's advice first.

Tying off

Skin tags can be strangled by tying dental floss or thread securely around the root of the stalk. This chokes off the blood supply and the tag will almost certainly fall off within a few days.

Natural remedies

Try blending castor oil and bicarbonate of soda into a paste and applying it three times a day. This should make the skin tag dry up within a few days. Tea tree oil or apple cider vinegar can also be effective if applied two to three times a day.

Permanent blemishes

Dermatosen Papulosa Nigra predominantly affects people with Black or Asian skins. It is characterised by dark, raised blemishes on the cheeks, forehead, neck and torso. The blemishes can sometimes become scaly. It is genetic, and harmless, so there is rarely a medical reason to treat. However, cosmetic treatments are available.

Seborrheic Keratosen is a variant of Dermatosen Papulosa Nigra, except that the spots may be lighter in colour. This mostly affects those people with fair skins. Both conditions are adult-onset, and the growths are benign, and can vary from pin-dots to up to an inch across.

Milia are caused by a build-up of dead skin cells that then become trapped under the skin, resulting in scatterings of small, white lumps, usually around the face and nose. Up to 50 per cent of all newborn babies have Milia, but in their case, it is caused by immature sebaceous glands, and goes away by itself, without any intervention. For adults, the suspected causes include sun damage, the over-use of topical steroids and dermabrasion. The spots are 1–2 mm in size, and are dome-shaped. All three conditions are painless, but can be unsightly.

£££ Cosmetic procedures

Dermatosen Papulosa Nigra and Seborrheic Keratosen can be treated in a variety of ways.

Freezing

The blemishes can be frozen off using liquid nitrogen. This procedure carries the risk of permanent scarring (including the formation of keloids – see page 60) which can be quite disfiguring and notoriously difficult to remove.

Scraping

The blemishes can also be scraped off with a scalpel, following the application of a topical local anaesthetic. Again, scarring is a risk.

Laser treatment

There has also been some success with laser treatment, particulary with the Nd:Yag laser. Risk of scarring is minimal.

Costs for laser treatment range from £500 to £1000 per session.

Chemical peels and microdermabrasion

Chemical peels (see page 23) can help to slough off the dead skin cells present in Milia and encourage new, healthy skin to grow.

Microdermabrasion (see page 31) can also be effective in clearing up mature skin affected by Milia.

Costs for chemical peels and microdermabrasion begin at around £60.

Permanent blemishes

££ Salon and make-up counter

AHAs and Retin-A

Alpha-hydroxy acids (AHAs) (page 24) and Retin-A (Tretinoin) (page 25) can be effective in treating all three conditions, though if you have darker skin you should be careful when using such products, as they have a potential to scar. Try AHAs made from lactic (milk) acid or malic (derived from apples and pears) acid, as these appear to be less damaging. Because Milia develop at the subcutaneous level, Retin-A can be helpful in treating it as it thickens the upper layers of skin.

£ Lifestyle and natural remedies

As Dermatosen Papulosa Nigra and Seborrheic Keratosen are believed to be genetic and are associated with ageing, there are no lifestyle changes that can offset their development or mitigate their appearance.

Avoid ...

Milia, on the other hand are possibly triggered by lifestyle factors, so avoid direct sunlight, harsh skin treatments and steroids. This could help to prevent them, or prevent their reappearance following successful treatment.

Razor bumps

Razor bumps are also known as "shaving bumps" or pseudofolliculitis barbae. They are the result of ingrown hairs that trigger a reaction in the skin and cause inflammation and even infection. The resultant raised lumps can turn red and, if bacteria is present, end up looking like an acne rash. People with curly hair are particularly susceptible, as curly hair is more prone to turn back into the hair follicle. If left untreated, razor bumps can be very unsightly and painful, and can even lead to the development of keloids (see pages 60 and 93).

The condition is generally caused and aggravated by shaving. It can occur in women as well as men, though men are predominantly affected. A good shaving routine can make all the difference, but persistent razor bumps can be effectively treated once they develop.

£££ Cosmetic procedures

Laser treatment

Laser treatment, using a Nd:YAG laser, has had encouraging results in the treatment of razor bumps, but be prepared for up to 12 sessions, spaced at several weeks' interval.

Drawbacks include discomfort and potential for scarring. Laser treatment does not provide a permanent solution, though it is a long-term one.

Costs for laser treatment start at £1000 per session.

££ Salon and make-up counter

Depilation creams

"Chemical shaving" using depilation creams is a popular means of by-passing razor-shaving because it avoids razor bumps. Depilation creams contain calcium thioglycolate, which weakens the hair so that it can be scraped off with ease.

However, it can irritate and even burn skin if left on longer than advised, and for this reason, it is usually not recommended for facial use.

Glycolic acid

You can also use a moisturiser containing glycolic acid (an AHA or fruit acid) at night. The glycolic acid helps the skin to slough off dead skin cells, which should help rid you of irritating bumps and keep the skin vibrant and healthy.

£ Lifestyle and natural remedies

Stop shaving

The best way to eliminate razor bumps is to stop shaving, at least for three to four weeks, therefore allowing the ingrown hairs to grow out properly. Many men find that having a beard is preferable to the discomfort and embarrassment of razor bumps.

Good shaving routine

However, if you prefer the clean-shaven look, then you need to develop a good shaving routine. First of all, never shave immediately after you wake up in the morning, as your skin is much more likely to be puffy from sleep. Wait ten minutes – that should be sufficient. Next, warm up your skin, either by taking a hot shower, or applying a warm washcloth, for at least five minutes. This softens skin, opens pores and, most importantly, softens the hairs that are about to be shaved.

A moisturising cleanser or gentle facial scrub will keep skin scrupulously clean, so try to make time for this before every shave. Then apply a moisturising shaving gel and, using a single-blade rather than multi-blade razor, shave using long, smooth strokes. Never shave against the grain, as cutting hairs the wrong way encourages them to curl back into the follicle. And keep the blade clean, rinsing thoroughly between strokes, and washing and sterilising between shaves.

Finally, rinse well, and apply an astringent after-shave or tea-tree oil to prevent infection. Shaving on alternate days, rather than every day, is another good tip for preventing razor bumps.

Face

It used to be that you had to live with the face you were born with. But as we've already seen in the previous chapter, there are now various ways to put the brakes on many of the symptoms of ageing. You can also alleviate the things about yourself that you're not so happy with – from under-eye circles to sticking-out ears. And not all of them involve an overnight stay at a clinic.

If you are considering a facial upgrade, remember that no amount of surgery will turn you into another person – but a great makeover can turn you into a very good version of yourself.

Eyes

Your eyes reveal how you are feeling – both physically and emotionally. No other feature makes such an impact.

There are a few simple things you can do to ensure that your eyes always look their best. Good quality, regular sleep is an absolute essential, because tiredness shows first in your eyes. No amount of clever make-up or cucumber eye patches will make up for late nights and early rises. Good diet is important too. Fresh produce, pure water and wholegrains all ensure that eyes remain clear and bright.

Make-up helps, so it's worth spending time with a make-up expert who can give you good advice about the best products to use for your eye shape and colour.

Always take time to cleanse the eye area thoroughly before you go to bed. After cleansing, dab a light eye-cream on with your ring finger (the weakest of your fingers) to ensure that you don't pull at the delicate skin of the eye area. Be careful not to put cream directly onto your eyelids, or they will become puffy.

Consult a good optician If you think you need glasses or contact lenses, as a lifetime of squinting will leave you lined and permanently frowning. If you work at a VDU screen, turn down the brightness and take regular screen breaks, as too much screen-time gives you red eyes and damages your vision. Similarly, give your eyes a rest from any kind of close work – from embroidery to reading – or you could damage them.

Puffy eyes

The skin of the eyelids is very thin and consequently very sensitive. The eyelids can become puffy for a number of reasons, including too much to drink the night before, fluid retention (due to too much salt in the diet), hayfever, hormonal changes, crying and lack of sleep. However, if the puffiness persists and is accompanied by pain and/or blurred vision, consult your GP or an eye specialist.

If your eyes become so puffy that you cannot comfortably close your eyes, you must seek medical guidance as quickly as possible, as there may be a medical condition underlying your problem.

£££ Cosmetic procedures

Puffy eyes are caused by fluid and there is therefore no appropriate surgical solution.

££ Salon and make-up counter

Eye creams

Soothing eye creams can help reduce inflammation and return eyes to their natural contours. Look for products containing aloe vera or vitamin E and always apply sparingly – too much eye cream can actually contribute to the problem in the first place.

101

Antihistamines

If your problem is caused by allergies, then anti-histamines should reduce eye puffiness and discomfort. These are available over-the-counter at most chemists.

£ Lifestyle and natural remedies

Sleep

Puffy eyes can be helped by getting plenty of sleep, especially when the head is elevated by a pillow.

Water

You can also reduce puffiness by drinking plenty of water to flush out toxins and by reducing your intake of salt and processed foods. Where possible, eat fruit, vegetables and wholegrains. Splashing the eyes with cold water helps to combat puffiness and tightens pores too.

Natural remedies

Home-made remedies include putting chilled slices of cucumber or cotton pads soaked in rosewater on your eyes for around ten minutes. You can also use chilled, used tea-bags or slices of Granny Smith apple. Both contain tannin, which is a natural anti-inflammatory. Finally, gentle massage round the eye area can improve lymphatic drainage, giving the eyelids a firmer appearance.

Hooded eyes

The "hood" of the eye covers, or partially covers, the eyelid. Hooded eyes can make you look weary or even sinister. They are generally hereditary or can develop with age, when fatty tissue begins to sag.

£££ Cosmetic procedures

Eyelid lift

An eyelid lift (or Blepharoplasty) is one of the most popular cosmetic surgery procedures in the world. It opens up the eyes and instantly rejuvenates the face.

If you opt for surgery, you should inform your surgeon of any eye problems you have, because these might disqualify you from surgery. The procedure usually involves a local anaesthetic. An incision is made in the upper eyelid, where it naturally creases, so that the scar will be discreet. Excess tissue and fat is then removed and the incision sutured, sometimes with dissolving stitches.

If there is excess skin, the surgeon might trim it, although they tend to err on the side of caution in this situation because too little skin is far worse than too much.

Bruising and swelling are common after-effects, but these are usually reduced within a few days through the regular application of ice-packs. You will probably be advised to sleep as upright as possible to ensure that the eyes drain properly at night.

You are also quite likely to be prescribed prophylactic antibiotics and eye ointment, to remove the risk of eye infection.

People often find it difficult to shut their eyes properly after this operation because of excessive tightness in the skin. This should subside within a few days. Eye drops are advised to treat the inevitable dryness of the eyes. Total recovery can take up to 12 weeks, though you can apply concealer within that time.

Costs range from £2500 to £5000.

££ Salon and make-up counter

There are no magical products available to treat this condition. However that is why make-up was invented!

Disguise hooded eyes

If you don't want to undergo surgery, then you can try using make-up to disguise your hooded lids. Choose a pale eyeshadow to begin with, a highlighter shade such as eau-de-nil, and apply from just above the upper lash line to the brow bone.

Next, apply a touch of shimmer eyeshadow to the lower eyelid. This will help to open up your eyes and will give a flash of brightness when you blink.

After this apply a mid-shade to the area above the lower eyelid. Finally, apply contour shade to the outer half of the eyelid, up to the brow bone, and under the lower lash line. Or you could use eyeliner under the lower lash line, extending it slightly beyond the outer edge of the eye. This will sweep the eye upwards, reducing the impact of the hooded lids.

£ Lifestyle and natural remedies

Don't exacerbate hooded eyelids by allowing the eyes to get puffy. And so get plenty of sleep, avoid too much alcohol, and drink plenty of water.

Under-eye bags

Bags under the eyes are a common symptom of tiredness. If they are severe, they can make you look older than you are. General causes include genetic predisposition, the ageing process and fluid retention. Sinus infection or allergies can also make under-eye bags worse, so consult your GP if you think this is the case.

£££ Cosmetic procedures

Eyelid lift

An eyelid lift is the recommended treatment for bags under the eyes. This involves a local anaesthetic and eyeball protection (see under "eyelid lift" page 103). In the case of eye bags the surgeon makes an incision inside the eyelid and then removes the fatty tissue. If there is excess skin, an incision is made just below the lash line along to the eye's outer edge and the skin is trimmed.

Skin can be resurfaced using a CO_2 laser about two or three weeks after surgery to remove any wrinkles. (For the recovery process and side-effects please refer to page 103).

Costs range from £2500 to £5000.

Fillers

Injectable line fillers such as Restylane and Juvederm are less invasive. They give the bags a smoother contour and make them less unsightly.

The effects last for nine months or so, after which the treatment needs repeated. Numbness is the main side-effect, but this gradually fades.

Costs begin at £250 per session.

££ Salon and make-up counter

Haemorrhoid cream

Haemorrhoid cream is one of the most popular fixes for under-eye bags. It's often used by models before a big shoot when they are trying to cover up the after-effects of the previous night's partying.

Cooling agents

Cooling, anti-inflammatory agents such as tea-bags, sliced apples and cucumber can also be effective (see also page 102).

£ Lifestyle

You can't cure eyebags if you are just naturally predisposed to them, but you can ensure you don't make them worse.

Get enough sleep, keep hydrated and don't overdo the partying!

Dark under-eye circles

Dark circles under the eyes are caused by a thinning of the skin, which in turn makes the bluish-red blood vessels beneath more visible.

Dark circles can make your face appear tired and prematurely aged. Dark circles on dark skins can be a result of over-pigmentation, and require a different approach from treatments recommended for fair skins.

£££ Cosmetic procedures

Laser treatment

Laser treatment vaporises the blood vessels and so reduces the darkness of the under-eye circle. This is only recommended for fair-skinned people, as lasers can reduce skin pigmentation in darker skins.

Costs for this procedure start from £1000.

££ Salon and make-up counter

Skin lightening agents

If you have darker skin then skin-lightening agents containing hydroquinone or the gentler kojic acid can help to reduce under-eye circles.

Creams

Products containing vitamins C, E and retinol have had

some positive results on all skins. Some people find that creams containing vitamin K can help, but there is less anecdotal evidence for this.

Cover up

You can cover up with concealer, but choose a pink shade, as white shades can make the dark skin appear grey. Pat on concealer after applying foundation. If you have sensitive skin and are prone to allergies, choose hypoallergenic cosmetics and avoid AHAs and glycolic acid, which can irritate thin, sensitive skin.

Special light-reflective concealers are also available, made especially for the area under the eye, and can be very effective.

£ Lifestyle and natural remedies

Get enough sleep

Lack of sleep is often said to make dark circles under the eye look much worse, so it is important to get plenty of sleep (8 hours per night is recommended).

Drink water

Keeping hydrated is important for all sorts of reasons, so it will do no harm to drink plenty of water to help to mitigate the appearance of dark circles.

Over-plucked and damaged eyebrows

Pencil thin eyebrows were popular in the 1970s, but not any more. They can make the face look severe and slightly expressionless.

Over-plucking is easy to do but very difficult to undo. The golden rule is never to pluck what you cannot live without, as you cannot be sure the plucked hair will grow back. Sometimes hair follicles can be so damaged by plucking that they cease to produce hairs.

£££ Cosmetic procedures

Eyebrow transplant

Chemotherapy, radiation treatment and physical trauma such as burns and facial injuries can damage the hair follicles to the extent that hair growth is no longer possible. This can leave you with no eyebrows or very sparse ones. In these cases, an eyebrow transplant is probably the only way to restore a natural look.

Eyebrow transplant surgery is an extremely specialised area, so be prepared for a long and difficult search for an appropriate surgeon.

There are two types of transplant:

- single hairs to the incision site or
- strips or flaps of hair, skin and underlying tissue to the incision site.

Single hair transplants usually result in a more defined

eyebrow. They use fine rather than coarse hair from the scalp (usually from the back of the head). This procedure requires a long time in surgery, or a series of procedures.

Flap transplants can be done in a single procedure. A flap is removed from the temple area in front of the ear and is then moved to the incision site while still attached to the underlying blood supply.

The flap is then tunnelled subcutaneously to the site until it "takes", and is nurtured by the local blood vessel system. If the transplant is successful, the patient must be prepared to "train" the new hair into the shape of an eyebrow using a small, mascara-like brush and gel and trim because the new hair will grow longer and faster than eyebrow hair.

Costs begin at around £2000.

Permanent and semi-permanent make-up

Eyebrows which are sparse or missing can be tattooed on. Finding a reputable practitioner is the most important factor. There are a lot of flashy websites out there but a personal recommendation and seeing some of the actual work the practitioner has done is the only way to proceed.

Eyebrow tattoos are usually done gradually and can be spaced out over a few weeks. The effect can last for several years but to keep looking fresh might need to be looked at again after around 12 to 18 months.

When it goes wrong, the fading process can leave eyebrows looking patchy and odd. Natural sagging of the skin can also affect how a tattooed brow ends up looking. Scarring is possible from the procedure as is an allergic reaction to the pigments used.

And there is the possibility that you will not like what has been done and it is not then easily removed. You can wait ten years or so for it to fade or pay from £175 to have another practitioner try to correct it.

This procedure can cost from £500.

££ Salon and make-up counter

Rogaine
It is difficult to speed up hair regrowth and impossible to stimulate growth once the follicle has died. There is, however, a product called Rogaine, that some people think is effective at stimulating hair growth. It was originally marketed at men, but there is now a version targeted specifically at women. Use with caution – this product must not get into your eyes.

Castor oil
Castor oil is an age-old "cure" for stunted hair growth that works for some but not others. Inexpensive so worth a try.

Stencilling kit
While you are waiting for new hairs to grow, you could try out an eyebrow stencilling kit. The stencil helps you to

fill in the eyebrow shape with the brow colour. Blend the colour in with the brushes until you have a soft, natural look. The fixative keeps it all in place until make-up removal time.

The added bonus of the stencil kit is that it also gives you a template for plucking your eyebrows. Stick to the template and you won't over-pluck again.

£ Lifestyle and natural remedies

Correct plucking

If you must pluck, then do a little regularly rather than a once-a-month binge where you are tempted to overdo it. Always err on the side of caution, use good quality, clean tweezers and work in a good light. Alternatively, you could have your eyebrows waxed or plucked at a salon. This will give you nice brows and a template to work from in future.

Threading is probably the most effective way of removing eyebrow hair. This Middle Eastern beauty treatment involves the use of a twisted thread to catch and remove all outlying hairs. A skilled practitioner can achieve very good, natural looking results. Threading also slows down regrowth because even tiny hairs are pulled out by the root.

Sparse eyelashes

Stubby, sparse lashes can be caused by pulling at eyelashes (perhaps a nervous habit) or overusing false eyelashes. In most cases, eyelashes grow back – unless the follicle has died.

£££ Cosmetic procedures

Eyelash restoration

Eyelash restoration is a very specialised field. Eyelash hairs are imported, one at a time, to give eyes a more natural look.

Following the procedure, the new hair must be "trained" to behave like eyelash hair, and your eyes might feel itchy. Avoid scratching, as this can dislodge the newly transplanted hairs and cause infection. Special spectacles can be prescribed to discourage scratching.

Costs start at £1500 per eye.

Permanent and semi-permanent make-up

See page 111 for eyebrow tattooing. The procedure and possible side-effects are similar, but obviously the eyelid is an even more delicate area. A tattoo gun is not used for this process.

The tattoo will aim to give the appearance of many lashes, to thicken sparsh lashes or give definition to eyes that have lost all their lashes.

Bruising and swelling can last three days to a week

following the procedure and there is risk of infection and allergic reaction. Costs start at around £350.

££ Salon and make-up counter

False eyelashes

False eyelashes are both a solution to and a cause of sparse lashes. Remove with great care. Eyelash glue can sometimes contain formaldehyde, and should therefore be avoided. This chemical can cause eye and skin problems.

Eyelash conditioners

Eyelash conditioners are a possible treatment, but make sure that they don't contain the active ingredient bimatoprost. This is a variant on a drug used to treat glaucoma and it can cause serious side-effects such as potential loss of sight, vision damage and changes to the colour of the iris.

Many eyelash conditioners have been reformulated since the glaucoma drug controversy came to light, but check carefully before using.

£ Lifestyle and natural remedies

Good health and personal care are key to keeping eyelashes lush. Avoid stress and get enough sleep.

Vaseline and olive oil are worth trying – although keep them away from your eyelids, or they might make them puffy.

Facial hair

Every woman has some facial hair. In children, it is usually soft, fine and fair. But from puberty onwards, it can become darker, coarser and more noticeable.

Genetic predisposition is a major cause as is ageing, and the natural hormonal changes that go with it.

Excess facial hair can be a symptom of an underlying medical problem such as Polycystic Ovary Syndrome (PCOS), which is a very treatable condition.

If you feel that your facial hair growth is excessive, you should consult your GP and rule out any medical explanation before proceeding with treatment

£££ Cosmetic procedures

Laser therapy

Laser therapy slows rather than stops hair growth, but it is worth investigating if you have stubborn and excessive facial hair.

Some people find it uncomfortable, while others find it painful. One side-effect can be scarring – particularly in darker skins.

Costs begin around £50 per session (for an upper lip, for example) though treatment can potentially cost several hundred pounds if repeat sessions are required.

Electrolysis

Electrolysis involves the insertion of a sterile needle into the hair follicle, where it discharges an electrical current. This effectively burns the hair off at the root, and in theory kills the follicle. It doesn't always work and since each hair follicle must be treated individually, it takes multiple treatments over many months. Some people find it uncomfortable, while others find it very painful.

Possible side-effects of electrolysis are scarring and changes in pigmentation, and, in some cases, infection.

Electrolysis costs from £20 per session of 15–20 minutes.

££ Salon and make-up counter

Waxing or sugaring

Waxing or sugaring is where hairs are removed by the root, by applying a thick sticky substance to the skin. A strip of material is placed on top of that and this material is then torn off, removing wax and – hopefully – all the unwanted hair.

Both are popular methods of getting rid of facial hair. They require a firm, steady hand and a bit of courage! For best results, pull the cotton strip away against the direction of hair growth.

You can also have these two treatments done at a salon, although this can be quite expensive if you want regular de-fuzzing.

Results last two to three weeks at the most.

Depilation cream

Depilation creams (see page 96) are effective at removing hairs but can irritate the skin if left on for too long, or if your skin is sensitive.

Results last two to three weeks at the most.

Bleaching

Bleaching is another way to minimise the appearance of facial hair by lightening it. Bleaching is only effective on short, fine hair and lasts only as long as it takes for the hair to grow enough to show its dark roots. Also, as it contains hydrogen peroxide it can irritate the skin to the extent of causing severe redness and blistering. You're best to do a patch test first.

£ Lifestyle and natural remedies

Natural method

If you don't like chemical treatments, try blending two teaspoonfuls of lemon juice (a known lightening agent) with two dessertspoonfuls of honey. Apply to hair and leave for ten to fifteen minutes before washing away.

Repeat this process once a week and it should remove some hairs and slow down growth

Plucking

Plucking is a reasonable method for occasional facial hairs, but it's not recommended for larger areas of facial hair – unless you're a masochist!

Shaving

Shaving is a quick fix, but you'll have stubble within a day or so. The ends of hairs will become sharp and stubbly. This might actually end up being worse than the longer, softer hairs you removed.

Thin lips

Thin lips are something you are born with, or tend to develop as part of the ageing process once collagen production decreases. They can make faces look rather severe.

There are a host of solutions on offer – some more successful than others.

£££ Cosmetic procedures

Lip fillers

Lip fillers are becoming increasingly popular and affordable.

The procedure takes around 30 minutes and includes the application of a topical, local anaesthetic. Lips can be injected with hyaluronic acid. This occurs naturally in the skin and joints and works by binding with water molecules to give lips a plumper, fuller appearance.

Bovine- or human-derived collagen is another injectable substance. Bovine-derived collagen has a slight allergy risk, so take an allergy test before the procedure. Human-derived collagen has no allergy risk.

Injections generally have no side-effects apart from a couple of days of swelling, though there is a minor risk of infection. The fullness lasts from four to six months, depending on how long it takes the body to break up and absorb the injected materials.

Fat injection

Lips can also be injected with the fat removed (via liposuction) from your own buttocks. There is little risk of rejection, as the injected material is your own. However, there is the risk of a scar where the fat was harvested, and results are not permanent.

Fillers cost around £300 per syringe, though using your own fat increases the price range from £1500 to £2000.

Lip implants

If you seek a permanent fix then you might want to consider lip implants. Before you do this, you are strongly advised to try out the non-permanent augmentations first, to see the shape and size that suits your lips.

The operation takes around an hour and includes a local anaesthetic. Two incisions are made at the outer corners of the lips. A tunnel is then made between the incisions and the implant is inserted. Finally, the incisions are sutured.

Implants are generally made of three materials.
- GORE-TEX – the same material used to make rain jackets – is a popular choice because it is porous and lip tissue can therefore grow through it. This creates a more natural effect. Apparently, it can also feel rather stiff.
- Softform Lip implants are tubular, which creates a soft result.
- AlloDerm is made from human tissue and gives the most natural look and feel of all.

Whenever you import a foreign body into human tissues, there is a risk of rejection, infection, and migration of the implants. This is also the case with lip implants. There can also be some rigidity.

Costs can begin at around £800 per lip.

Semi-permanent make-up

Semi-permanent make-up can be a preferable alternative to lip fillers and implants which can result in allergic reactions and rejection. Lips can be coloured and shaded to look plumper or more even.

Consider carefully before you decide that a permanent lip liner or lip blush from a tattoo will be the answer to the problem of thin lips as the risks and side-effects that can occur as a result of eyebrow and eyelash tattoos (see pages 111 and 114) apply to lip tattoos also.

Costs start at around £400.

££ Salon and make-up counter

Lip plumpers

Lip plumpers provide a temporary boost to thin lips. Some claim to boost collagen production and suggest that the effect will be more long-lived.

Lip plumpers generally work either by attracting water molecules (which gives lips a fuller, plumper look) or by including an irritant, such as cinnamon, wintergreen or peppermint (which makes lips look fuller and redder).

Some lip plumpers also include hyaluronic acid, a natural plumping agent.

£ Lifestyle and natural remedies

Avoid ...
Smoking leads to lines round your mouth and will dry out even the most luscious of lips – so stop now.

Exfoliate
A weekly exfoliation using soft toothbrush will help to give your lips a healthy pinkness, while a dab (but don't overdo it) of cinnamon oil will do much the same work as a commercial lip plumper.

Make-up
You can also use make-up to great effect.

First of all, avoid dark lipsticks and lip pencils, which can make even bee-stung lips look thinner and more severe.

Begin by covering the lips in your usual foundation, then apply a pale or nude lipliner around the outer edge of your lips. Some make-up artists think this looks instantly fake, but it's worth trying out. Always be sure to smudge the lipliner, as a distinct line only draws attention to your lips' actual contours.

Next, apply your usual lipstick, then dab highlighter in the bow of the lips, or the centre of the lower lip, to

Thin lips

open up the area, making it appear broader.

Try gold or silver highlighter, depending on your colouring. The shimmery effect brings in more light, increasing the volumising effect.

Finally, coat with lipgloss. Lipgloss attracts light to make the lips appear more luscious.

Receding chin

A receding chin can throw off the whole balance of a face, making the nose appear more prominent and the jowls fleshy. It can be caused by a misalignment of the lower jaw due to:

- a congenital condition
- the upper and lower jaws growing at uneven rates
- physical trauma.

This condition can also make it difficult to chew, speak and even breathe, and it can be a source of considerable pain and discomfort.

A receding chin can also be a cosmetic flaw that causes no pain but severely diminishes personal confidence.

There are surgical treatments for both conditions, and a few handy tricks to help out too.

£££ Cosmetic procedures

Orthognathic surgery

Orthognathic surgery is required for treatment of a misaligned lower jaw.

Retrognathia (or receding lower jaw) can also cause a significant overbite, and surgery is recommended when orthodontic treatment alone cannot correct the problem.

Orthognathic surgery is a big commitment, as full results take a minimum of two years, and the pre- and after-care is significant.

Receding chin

Work begins with pre-surgical orthodontics, so that the teeth fit together properly post-surgery. This can require the wearing of braces for up to two years. Progress is monitored on an ongoing basis, using X-rays and dental moulds.

When your orthodontist thinks you are ready, you then proceed to surgery. You will be admitted to hospital on an in-patient basis after extensive consultation with your surgeon.

You will be given a general anaesthetic before the operation, which can take several hours, depending on the extent of work required. Orthognathic surgery is usually very successful, and the results are predictable.

During the operation, the jaw might be separated in more than one place and bone is sometimes added to achieve the required length. Once the jaw is aligned, a portion of the chin bone is brought forward to achieve a better profile. The parts of the jaw and the chin bone are then fixed in place with plates and screws.

You will probably stay in hospital for a few days after the operation. Your diet will be liquid only because your jaws will be held rigid to assist healing. The initial recovery period is around six weeks. During this time the swelling and bruising should recede, and you might be prescribed prophylactic antibiotics and anti-inflammatory painkillers. A full recovery – including the knitting of the tissue – can take up to a year.

As with all major operations risk of infection is high,

so be rigorous about your oral hygiene and attend all subsequent out-patient appointments with your surgeon and dentist.

After the operation your orthodontist will want to fine-tune your teeth, so you might have to wear braces for a further year or so.

If post-operative problems such as chronic pain or limited movement persist, you might need further treatment. Any damage to fillings and bridgework that happened during the operation will be sorted out in the months following surgery.

The results of this procedure can be transformative – not just to the appearance but also to your health and general wellbeing.

Retrognathia is usually conducted following a clinical referral, so costs can be met on the NHS.

Chin implants

If your receding chin is not as a result of misalignment, chin implants are a popular solution.

Implants can be made of silicone or a porous substance such as ePTFE, and can be trimmed to fit by your surgeon. A local anaesthetic is applied topically before an incision is made, either beneath the chin or inside the mouth. A small pouch is created immediately in front of the chin bone and the implant is inserted here. Alternatively, the implant can be affixed to tissue or bone.

The procedure should take around an hour. After-effects include swelling and bruising and a temporary numbness. If the incision was made within the mouth then you'll be on a liquid diet for a while. Oral hygiene is essential.

A tape or chin strap can be used to hold the implant in place during the swelling phase, though this carries a longer term risk of migration and infection.

Costs for this procedure vary from £2000 to £3000.

Injectable fillers

Injectable fillers (such as calcium hydroxylapatite) are non-permanent, but they're a good way of assessing whether you would suit an implant. They are usually administered in two 15-minute sessions. The results are generally subtle, but they can improve a weak profile.

This treatment can last up to two years, by which time the material has been broken up and reabsorbed by the body.

Fillers cost from £300 per syringe.

££ Salon and make-up counter

Haircut

Avoid a chin-length haircut because this draws the eye to the chin area. Try a longer or shorter haircut with layering or perming – these styles create volume, which can make a receding chin less noticeable. Men have the option of growing a beard.

Make-up

Women can use make-up to disguise a receding chin. Apply bronzer or shading powder to the area beneath the jawline. Blend this in well to avoid a tide-mark. Then apply highlighter to the top of the chin, to bring it forward. Attention to eye make-up can draw people's attention upwards, making a slightly receding chin almost invisible to the casual observer.

£ Lifestyle and natural remedies

Posture

If you improve your posture, then you'll improve your profile. Holding your head high will make a weak chin look more prominent and draw attention away from the nose. It will also lengthen the neck, reducing the appearance of jowls.

Prominent ears

Prominent or "bar" ears can be a terrible source of teasing for young children and can make adults feel cripplingly self-conscious. The definition of prominent ears is that they protrude more than 40 degrees from the side of the head when viewed from above,

Many people learn to live with prominent ears. Many don't – and opt for surgery.

Early intervention at newborn stage can correct ear problems and remove the need for surgery later.

Other ear conditions, such as "Stahl's bat" or pointed ears, "lop ear" (where the upper half of the ear flops over) and "rim kinks" (where there are bumps and kinks in the rim of the upper ear) can also be treated either non-surgically when very young, or surgically when full-grown.

£££ Cosmetic procedures

Otoplasty

Otoplasty ("pinning" the ears back) is the most common paediatric cosmetic surgery procedure in the UK. It cannot be performed before the age of five, as the ear is still too soft and malleable. It can also be conducted very successfully on adults.

A local or general anaesthetic is administered, and incisions are then made at the back of the ear. If incisions have to be made at the front, they will be made in naturally existing folds, to minimise scarring.

During the operation the cartilage is folded back towards the ear to make it less prominent. In some cases it might have to be trimmed and moulded into shape before folding. Finally, the incisions are sutured, often with dissolving stitches. The operation usually lasts around 90 minutes,

You usually have to wear a bandage for a week or so after the operation. You are advised to wear a headband at night for a further six weeks. This keeps the ear folds in place and minimises the risk of the ear catching on anything.

You must avoid contact sports during this recovery period.

This is a very common operation, so risks are quite small but they include loss of sensation on the skin of the ear, bleeding and infection. Serious infection can lead to cartilage damage, which could mean further, corrective surgery, so attend all follow-up appointments and act on after-care advice.

Results are visible immediately, though you will be advised to expect improvement rather than transformation

Ear deformities such as "Stahl's Bat" can also be successfully treated through otoplasty.

Costs for this procedure range from £1500 to £3000.

££ Salon and make-up counter

Neonatal moulding

Neonatal moulding is another option for prominent ears.

In neonatal moulding a soft, corrective splint is inserted into the gully of the ear to create the preferred shape.

Tape is then applied to pin the ear closer to the head, and the soft cartilage heals into that shape.

In newborn babies this process takes a few weeks. In three month old babies the process can take up to four months. It's best to do this procedure when babies are newborn, because they rarely move their heads, they can't remove the tape and their cartilage is soft and malleable.

This process isn't quite so easy for adults. Taped ears can be socially embarrassing, and the process can take up to a year before there are any positive results.

£ Lifestyle and natural remedies

There are no lifestyle choices that can help prominent ears.

Turkey neck

The neck and the hands are the biggest give-away when we are trying to look younger. For most of us, skincare stops at the jawline and the delicate skin of the neck and decolletage is neglected. In time, this makes for slack muscles, loose skin and crepey, "chicken-skin" texture.

The first step to preventing turkey neck is to include the neck in your daily skincare routine.

The second step is to cover up with sunscreen, just as you would your face. This will also guard against liver or age spots, which frequently pop up on neglected neck skin.

Finally, if you wear make-up, consider wearing it on your neck and decolletage too. This will give you a more natural, overall coverage. It will also protect your skin from UV rays and environmental pollutants, which can damage skin cells and cause them to age more rapidly.

£££ Cosmetic procedures

Neck lifts are often done in conjunction with a face and/ or brow lift. There are seven different types of procedure to help turkey neck.

Expect to pay between £3000 and £5000 for any kind of necklift procedure.

Platysmaplasty
Platysmaplasty tackles the problem of sagging skin

associated with neck muscles that have loosened with age.

The procedure begins with a local anaesthetic. The surgeon makes two incisions – one behind each ear – and then possibly a third, immediately under the chin. The neck muscles (or platysma) are then tightened or shortened and fixed in place with sutures. This procedure can be done endoscopically, using a tiny camera. This shortens the duration of the operation and reduces the risks and side-effects.

Cervicoplasty

Cervicoplasty is performed if the problem lies with loose skin. The procedure is the same as with platysmaplasty, except that it is the skin that is pulled taut and then trimmed and sutured. Patients are usually advised to wear a compression bandage for a week afterwards, to promote healing.

The immediate after-effects of both these procedures is swelling and bruising. The initial recovery period should last for about two weeks.

Avoid vigorous sports for around six weeks. Infection and bleeding are a risk after all major operations, so take due care during the recovery period.

Liposuction

Liposuction (see pages 35 and 85) is the recommended procedure for excess fat on the neck.

During this procedure the incision is usually made

beneath the chin. The operation should take around an hour. Liposuction can be done in conjunction with platysmaplasty or cervicoplasty, or even both.

Subcutaneous plastic sling

One recent innovation is the insertion of a subcutaneous plastic sling, made of GORE-TEX. The sling stretches from ear to ear. It tightens neck muscles and can be adjusted in future years in a quick follow-up procedure that involves the re-opening of the earlobe incisions and a tightening of the sling.

This procedure can sometimes cause infection and inflammation.

Threadlifts

Threadlifts (see page 34) are another option. They can be removed immediately if there are complications.

This procedure costs around £1500 per area treated.

Other treatments

The Titan laser uses infrared to stimulate collagen production, and has had some success in treating ageing necks. A series of treatments is required, and improvement may take a number of months.

Laser treatment costs from £500
Botox injections (see page 27) relax the neck muscles, thereby reducing the appearance of vertical bands.

Costs start from £300 per syringe.

Thermage is less invasive and can leave skin looking and feeling firmer and more youthful.

Costs start from £1500.

££ Salon and make-up counter

Creams

Look for creams containing intensely moisturising ingredients such as avocado oil and shea butter, and skin vitamins A, C and E.

Plant hormones and rice proteins or extracts also claim to have firming properties, and feature in some recommended neck creams.

Tretinoin, or Retin-A, is also effective, but is only available on prescription.

£ Lifestyle and natural remedies

Exercise

Vigorous exercise is great for overall skin tone.

Drink plenty of water and eat lots of vitamin C – both will help your skin.

Here's an exercise that will help to tighten your neck muscles:

Tilt the head backwards while still looking straight ahead. Do this slowly, count to ten, and then slowly bring your head back to the normal level. Repeat regularly. You'll be able to feel your muscles contract.

Nose imperfections

The nose is one of the most prominent facial features and as such, it is the one we fixate on if we think it is flawed. The shape of the nose is largely determined by genetic make-up, though abnormal growth patterns and injury can also knock it out of shape.

It's not surprising then that rhinoplasty or a "nose job" is one of the most popular cosmetic surgery procedures in the world. An over-large nose, flared nostrils, a bumpy or raised bridge and a rounded or drooping nose tip are just some of the issues that can obsess people.

£££ Cosmetic procedures

Rhinoplasty

If you feel that you can't live with your nose, then rhinoplasty is a hugely popular procedure. Many surgeons have extensive experience in this field, so it is relatively safe, and outcomes are generally predictable. A good surgeon will remain true to your ethnic origin and bone structure, so look carefully at a range of before and after pictures of patients they have worked on. Rhinoplasty can only be performed on adults because the nose continues to grow until at least the age of 13.

Surgery will give you an improved version of the nose you already have – not a completely new one. It's essential that you have realistic expectations.

Nose imperfections

The procedure takes around two to three hours and begins with the administration of a general anaesthetic. Incisions are either made inside the nose, or across the tissue that separates the nostrils. This is called the columella.

Skin and tissue are then separated and raised to allow access to the cartilage, which is reshaped, shaved down or even augmented to achieve the desired shape and profile.

The upper cartilage is "shaved" to even out a rounded or bumpy bridge or to reduce the nose's overall size. The septum – between the nostrils – can also be trimmed to size thereafter. The alar cartilage at the end of the nose can be moulded or even trimmed down to reduce a bulbous or drooping nose. Nostrils can be narrowed by cutting away tiny wedge-shaped areas of skin and tissue within the natural folds to minimise scarring. If the nose needs to be augmented, cartilage grafts can be taken from the ear or rib and used to build it up.

Once the shaping and re-sizing is complete, the skin and tissue are drawn back down into place. Internal tubes are inserted to act as splints, and these usually stay in place for around a week. External splints might also be necessary.

Bleeding is quite common after rhinoplasty, and you will probably be told not to blow your nose for several days afterwards, as the tissue needs time to settle down. Avoid contact sports for at least six weeks. Swelling and bruising last for two to three weeks. Swelling can also return intermittently for up to a year because this is approximately how long it takes for the nose to settle into its new shape.

Scarring is generally minimal.

Two serious complications can arise from rhinoplasty.

Eye injury can occur if the tear ducts become damaged during surgery, so ask about eye protection.

Meningitis is another possible complication, due to the nasal injuries that can occur during rhinoplasty. Symptoms include headaches, sensitivity to light and neck stiffness. You should be aware that adults sometimes present no symptoms at all initially.

Costs range from £4000 to £8000.

££ Salon and make-up counter

While there are no beauty products available that can change the shape of your nose, there are a few cosmetic tricks you and your hairdresser or beautician can use to disguise an imperfect nose.

Hairstyles

Avoid short or flat hairstyles, as they emphasise facial features. Opt instead for mid-length to long hairstyles, with plenty of soft volume. Wavy hair gives an impression of broadness to the face and therefore detracts attention from the nose.

Spectacles

Spectacles can also improve the appearance of a nose, so even if you don't need a prescription, a pair of flattering frames with clear glass lenses can give your looks a boost.

Make-up

Make-up is also helpful. Use bronzer to shade the sides of the nose and make it look smaller and finer. Blend as you go with a soft cosmetic brush.

Make the most of your eyes, using bright, dramatic colours. Close-set eyes create an emphasis on the nose, so follow these tips to create an effect of wide-set eyes. Begin by applying light eyeshadow at the inner corners of the eyes (from lash to brow) and extend coverage to two thirds of the lid area. Dab highlighter in the inner corner, to open up the eye. Apply darker shadow to the final third of eyelid area, sweeping up to the brow. Then apply highlighter to the brow bone.

Eyeliner should be heaviest at the outer edges, and extra coats of mascara can be added to outer lashes, to extend the sweep of the eye. Finally, extend eyebrows away from the nose by using a brow pencil.

£ Lifestyle and natural remedies

Bear in mind that although the nose on your face is very plain to you, it's probably no big deal to anybody else. The main thing you can do to get over self-consciousness is concentrate on all your good points, quit making negative comments about yourself and try develop your self-confidence.

Teeth

We associate perfect, white and even teeth with good health and youthfulness – and stained, damaged teeth with disease and old age.

Nothing is more off-putting than a brown smile riddled with holes, which is why lots of us are willing to pay to achieve white teeth.

A recent survey by the British Academy of Cosmetic Dentists found that a third of us are concerned about the look of our teeth, while one fifth of us are so ashamed that we don't smile in photos. But good teeth are not just aesthetically appealing. Women associate a nice smile with a warm personality, while men associate it with success. To maintain healthy teeth ensure that your general health is good and eat a diet rich in calcium (for building strong teeth) and phosphorous. Avoid fizzy drinks, which can leach phosphorous from the body.

To keep any problems to a minimum, brush twice daily with a good, fluoride toothpaste and replace your toothbrush every three to four months, or sooner if it's showing wear. You should also have regular check-ups with the dentist

Discoloured teeth

There are different causes of discolouration. The most common is the ageing process, when teeth gradually turn yellower or browner. Staining foods and drinks such as tea, coffee and red wine are also responsible for the discolouration of teeth. Tobacco – either chewed or smoked – also stains teeth.

Dental fluorosis, caused by the ingestion of excessive fluoride, can result in mottled, darkly stained teeth. It can occur in adults and in newborn babies whose mothers took too much fluoride during pregnancy. Tetracyline antibiotics can turn teeth a shade of grey – especially in young children, whose tooth enamel is not yet fully developed. It can also occur in newborn babies whose mothers took tetracycline during pregnancy.

Grey or pink teeth can also be the result of injury and even root canal treatment.

£££ Cosmetic procedures (dentistry)

Cosmetic dentistry is a huge growth area, and tooth whitening is one of the most requested procedures.

Ultrasonic cleaning

Ultrasonic cleaning is a gentle but very effective method of brightening teeth. It involves the use of a scaling tip that vibrates gently to dislodge plaque, tartar and even stains on the teeth, without damaging the enamel.

Enamel Microbrasion

Enamel Microbrasion removes dental fluorosis, and is a very safe treatment. A mixture of weak hydrochloric acid and silicone carbide particles is combined into a paste and rubbed onto the teeth. It removes staining in the enamel.

Bleaching

Bleaching is increasingly popular. It makes your teeth a few shades lighter. The treatment begins with a consultation with your dentist, who will take impressions of your teeth and gums.

First, a gum shield or protective gel is applied to the gums to stop them being damaged by the bleaching agent (usually hydrogen peroxide and/or carbamide). The bleaching agent is then applied via the rubber mould that was made from your teeth.

One or two treatments can be required. This is followed by a self-administered treatment at home, where the bleaching agent is applied to teeth (again via the rubber mould) during the night.

Costs begin at around £500 for the whole mouth.

Laser whitening

In laser whitening the laser activates the ingredients in the paste and make the process faster and more effective.

Laser whitening starts at £1000 for the whole mouth

After-effects of bleaching include sensitivity to cold, some gum discomfort and even white patches on the gum line. These should all disappear quite quickly. Avoid the bad habits that discoloured your teeth in the first place or you'll end up back where you started.

Veneers

If the discolouration is too bad to be treated with bleaching agents, then you could try veneers. These are super-thin covers – rather like artificial fingernails – that are glued directly over the front of your damaged teeth to achieve a clean, white smile. Veneers are usually made of porcelain or ceramic, though they can also be made of a composite material that is built up on the tooth directly. They are glued to the teeth using a resin cement. Because they tend to look rather startlingly white compared to the rest of your teeth it's a good idea to veneer several (if not all) of your teeth at the same time.

Veneers (particularly porcelain ones) can be brittle, and can cause problems such as overly enlarging the teeth if they are not properly prepared and applied. Therefore, choose your cosmetic dentist with care and insist on seeing before and after pictures of previous clients.

Veneers cost from around £175 per tooth.

££ Salon and make-up counter

There are lots of tooth whitening toothpastes and kits on the market, but be careful what you buy. If in doubt, read the label.

Avoid pumice, which is simply an abrasive. While it will remove some discolouration it will also damage your tooth enamel. This will in turn make your teeth weaker and even more vulnerable to staining.

Baking soda

Baking soda is a popular ingredient in whitening toothpastes and is perfectly safe. It won't give you stunningly white teeth, but it can be effective at stain removal. Use it as you would tooth powder or paste, and rinse afterwards.

Whitening strips

Whitening strips are plastic strips that are coated with a substance usually containing hydrogen peroxide. These strips must be placed on the teeth and left there for around 30 minutes. They can sometimes leave areas unwhitened.

Home bleaching kits

Home bleaching kits comprise a tray and a bleaching agent. However, these trays are not made to fit your particular teeth and can lead to leakage. Also, when applied to your gums, hydrogen peroxide can cause blisters and intense sensitivity. Bleaching should always be done by a professional dentist to ensure good, safe results.

Discoloured teeth

Electric toothbrushes

Electric toothbrushes can achieve up to 7000 brushstrokes a minute – much more than you could do yourself. Sonic toothbrushes have an extra cleaning action and give your teeth an even more rigorous brushing than ordinary electric toothbrushes.

£ Lifestyle and natural remedies

Regular brushing

Brush your teeth gently and thoroughly twice a day for at least two minutes to remove all plaque and residual foodstuffs. A dental hygienist will be happy to show you how.

If you're really committed to keeping your teeth white then avoid staining substances such as tea, coffee, fizzy drinks and red wine, and stop smoking.

Crooked teeth

Crooked teeth can result from gum disease, having too many teeth for the size of your mouth, excessive thumb or dummy sucking after the age of three years and facial injury – or they can be an inherited trait.

Crooked teeth can also be caused by a misalignment of the jaw. (Please refer to the "receding chin" section on page 125 for details of the surgical treatment for this.)

In the worst cases, crooked teeth can cause dental problems such as pain when chewing.

£££ Cosmetic procedures (dentistry)

Orthodontics

Orthodontics is the traditional way to correct crooked teeth. This is only suitable for people who have all their adult teeth and who don't have gum disease or tooth decay, as wearing braces can exacerbate both.

An orthodontist will examine your teeth and take X-rays so they can fully understand the problem. They might even recommend taking teeth out if overcrowding is contributing to the crookedness. Braces will then be custom-made to fit your mouth. These comprise brackets (made of ceramic, plastic or metal) that are glued to the front of your teeth and a wire that gradually pushes the teeth into the required shape. The wire will be pulled tighter at regular intervals. The treatment is painless and can be almost invisible if ceramic brackets are used.

Lingual braces are applied to the backs of the teeth, and are even harder to notice. This is a long-term treatment and the final result can take up to two years to achieve.

No matter what type of brace you choose, the orthodontist will probably recommend that you wear a retainer for several months after it has been taken out, to keep the teeth from moving back to their original position.

Oral hygiene is crucial. Your orthodontist will advise you on how to keep your teeth clean.

Costs range from £600 to £4000.

Invisalign braces

Invisalign braces are relatively new. They are clear plastic and are therefore virtually invisible. Like conventional braces, they force your teeth to gradually shift into a more optimum position. Invisalign braces are custom-made and are replaced every two weeks.

As with conventional braces, six-weekly appointments are necessary to ensure that teeth are moving as predicted. Invisalign braces are worn nearly all the time, and are only removed when you need to eat, drink or clean them. Conventional braces are worn all the time.

Costs start at around £2000.

Veneers

Veneers are a third option (see page 144).

Dental contouring

If the crookedness is only slight, it can be corrected with cosmetic dental contouring. This is relatively cheap and very quick compared to orthodontics. The dentist begins by taking X-rays to establish that there is enough bone between the areas of teeth pulp to proceed. A laser or sanding drill is then used to remove tiny layers of enamel, until the required shape is achieved. Abrasive strips can also be used between the teeth to create a smooth, polished appearance. You might need veneers (that are built up on the tooth) to finish off.

This method can also be effective for treating cracked, chipped or overlapping teeth, and it generally requires between one and three sessions of treatment.

Costs start at around £50 per tooth

££ Salon and make-up counter

There are no beauty products that can deal effectively with crooked teeth.

£ Lifestyle and natural remedies

There is little you can do to prevent crooked teeth. However, you can make the best of your teeth by cleaning them regularly, following a good diet and avoiding substances that can stain them.

Gummy smile

"Gumminess" or "gummy smile" is a condition where an excessive amount of gum is shown when you smile. This can make your teeth look small and your gums look very large, and can be one reason why so many of us avoid toothy smiles to the camera.

Gummy smile is often hereditary, but it can also be caused by chronic mouth breathing. This causes the gums to become dry and red and to grow over the teeth. Other causes include the side-effects of certain medications prescribed for epilepsy, orthodontic treatment and chronic teeth-grinding.

£££ Cosmetic procedures

Gum tissue removal

A gingivectomy is usually enough to eradicate minor gumminess. In this procedure excess gum tissue is removed under local anaesthetic with a scalpel. No stitches are required and gums usually heal within two weeks to reveal larger teeth and a more even gumline.

Excess tissue can also be removed with a laser, which can also cauterise the wounds by sealing off the blood vessels.

Radiosurgery is another option, and uses a 4MHz high frequency.

For more extensive gumminess, gum tissue can be

surgically lifted to achieve a higher, more aesthetically pleasing gumline. Some bone might also have to be removed.

This procedure requires sutures, which are removed after one or two weeks. Thereafter, full healing may take up to six weeks.

Cosmetic gum surgery costs between £150 to £300 per tooth.

Veneers

You might need veneers to finish off the treatment because the newly exposed teeth might not have full enamel coverage. This part of the procedure would have to wait until the end of the full recovery period.

Crowns

If grinding is the cause, then the teeth might have to be lengthened by applying crowns. Crowns or caps can be used to improve cracked or broken teeth as well as those worn down by chronic teeth grinding. However, crowns are only recommended when the tooth is too weak or reduced to support veneers, because they require the original, often healthy tooth to be partially removed.

The procedure begins with the administration of a local anaesthetic. The dental surgeon then reshapes the tooth and pares it down to accommodate a crown by using a dental drill called a "burr". An impression of the newly reduced tooth is taken and sent to a dental laboratory, where it is used to create a custom-made crown. This takes around three weeks. Meanwhile, you will be fitted with a temporary crown.

A crown can be made of porcelain or ceramic, or of a metal alloy fused to porcelain. Porcelain or ceramic-only crowns are advised for front teeth, as metal-based crowns will start to show through at the gumline after a number of years. When the crown is ready the temporary one will be removed, the surface of the original tooth roughened so as to bond well with the cement and the new crown affixed.

A good crown should last from ten to fifteen years if it is looked after.

A crown costs around £350.

Medication

Gumminess can be a side-effect of certain medication. If so, try another type or, if possible, come off it altogether. The gums will then recede to their normal position. If they don't then try some of the above strategies.

Coronally positional mucosal flap surgery

Finally, if a high lipline is the reason for gumminess, this can be remedied with a surgical procedure known as CPMF (coronally positional mucosal flap) surgery. It is a simple, usually successful treatment.

Once the local anaesthetic has been administered the gum tissue behind the upper lip is reattached, to inhibit the movement of the lip. Suitable candidates for this procedure must be able to close their mouths over their teeth, otherwise the operation will not produce desired results.

One of the common after-effects of CPMF surgery is a tighter upper lip.

High lipline surgery costs in the region of £800.

££ Salon and make-up counter

There are no beauty products available that can alleviate gumminess.

£ lifestyle

There are no lifestyle changes that you can make to alleviate gumminess.

Receding gums

Receding gums make the teeth appear longer and rather more spaced out. Causes can include ageing, lack of oral hygiene, and aggressive overbrushing over some years.

Gingivitis is the term used to describe inflamed (and possibly bleeding) gums. Check your toothbrush for a pinkish tinge after brushing. If you leave food particles stuck between your teeth they breed bacteria, which can lead to inflamed gums and, possibly, periodontal disease.

Periodontal disease can be very serious, because it can make your teeth loosen and fall out. It can also eat away at your bone structure so that you don't even have enough left to support dentures.

Other causes of gum recession include chronic teeth grinding, misaligned teeth, smoking or chewing tobacco and poor oral hygiene. Mouth jewellery, such as lip or tongue piercings, can also be a contributory factor.

Gum recession and gum disease can make your teeth very sensitive and sore. On a more serious level, they can be linked to conditions such as heart disease and diabetes, so check with your dentist and GP if you have any doubts.

£££ Cosmetic procedures (dentistry)

Desensitising agent

If your gums are sensitive, your dentist can treat them

with a desensitising agent such as a flouride gel. You will then be recommended to use a sensitive formula toothpaste on a regular basis. This will form a protective layer over your tooth if you don't rinse after brushing.

Night guard

If you grind your teeth at night, your dentist can provide you with a night guard.

Orthodontics

Misaligned teeth can be successfully treated through orthodontics (see page 147).

Debridement

If you want to deep clean your teeth, you could opt for a debridement, which usually takes place over four sessions. The hygienist cleans a quarter of your mouth at a time. Sometimes a local anaesthetic is administered before each treatment.

Debridement involves scaling (where plaque and tartar are manually scraped from the surface of the tooth), root planing (where the nooks and crannies that bacteria like to live in are smoothed away) and polishing (where the surface of the tooth is too sheer to harbour bacteria).

This deep clean can be repeated twice or even three times a year. It will not restore the receding gums, but it will ensure that your teeth are healthy and that the recession is stopped.

Debridement can cost around £150 per quadrant of the mouth.

Gum graft surgery

If gum recession is advanced, then gum graft surgery is an option. In this procedure, gum tissue is harvested from elsewhere in the mouth and used to patch over particularly badly exposed roots. Gum graft surgery will only be considered when the causes of the gum recession have been fully treated

A pedicle graft is common. In this procedure a flap of skin is lifted from a neighbouring tooth and used to patch up the root, while still attached to the original blood supply. The skin can also be taken from the roof of the mouth (the palate) and sutured in place. This will improve the look of the gumline.

Costs begin at around £300 per tooth.

££ Salon and make-up counter

There are no beauty products available that can alleviate receding gums.

£ Lifestyle and natural remedies

Brushing technique is important for prevention of gum disease, and in order not to exacerbate any existing symptoms of receding gums. A soft toothbrush is recommended for receding gums. Teeth should be brushed gently and in a circular, or up and down, motion, rather than side to side. Look online, some toothpaste manufacturers have posted videos to show you the correct brushing method. It's usually recommended to brush gently twice a day, for two minutes at a time. Those with receding gums could brush one extra time in the middle of the day too, one hour after food.

Flossing is also very important, as this will remove food particles and keep bacteria at bay. Regular check-ups with your dentist – perhaps every three months – will ensure that any potential problems will be spotted before they dig in.

De-sensitising toothpaste can soothe any pain from the condition, and using one designed specifically for gum health may also help prevent it occurring in the first place. There are mouthwashes that can help prevent gum disease too.

Avoid sugary snacks and fizzy drinks.

Smoking is a cause of gum disease, so if you smoke, please stop now.

Hair

We associate thick, lustrous hair with youth, vitality, fertility and beauty. And we associate thin, grey, lank hair with ageing, ill-health and misery.

We spend millions of pounds on our hair, and the phrase "bad hair day" has become synonymous with nothing going right for us.

On average, we have 100,000 hairs on our head, each with a lifespan of between two and seven years, and with an average growth rate of 12 cm a year.

Female hair grows more slowly than men's, but as we age, both sexes find that their hair growth rate slows and that there is less of it. By the age of 50, around half of all men have male pattern hair loss. By the time they reach menopause, some 40 per cent of women have female pattern hair loss. By the time we are in our 50s the melanin that causes hair pigment starts to fail, resulting in greying, increasingly colourless hair.

However, there are a whole host of products and treatments for every kind of hair problem, from lankness to hair loss.

Hair loss (men)

Male pattern baldness can begin as early as the late 20s, but usually becomes apparent in a thinning of the hair at the temples in the 30s or early 40s.

It is caused by dihydrotesterone, or DHT – a by-product of testosterone, the hormone responsible for a male's primary and secondary sexual characteristics. DHT makes hair follicles shrink and weaken, making growth cycles increasingly short and hairs increasingly thin (especially around the crown and temples) until eventually the follicles stop producing hairs altogether.

Male pattern baldness is hereditary and there is little you can do to prevent it, though stress, poor diet and illness can accelerate it.

There are other causes of hair loss in men, including a lack of iron in the diet (anaemia), severe stress, certain medications and fungal scalp infections.

If your hair loss does not conform to the typical male pattern of crown and temple thinning but instead is characterised by a patchiness overall, then it is worth consulting your GP to eliminate other possible causes.

Baldness is the butt of endless jokes, but it can be far from funny – especially if you're young.

It can cause a significant drop in self-confidence or even lead to depression because the perception is that it detracts from a man's physical attractiveness (although there are many women out there who strongly disagree!).

There are many treatments available for hair loss, but they don't work for everybody. The cure for male pattern baldness has not been invented yet so until it is, the best cure is to come to terms with it.

£££ Cosmetic procedures

Hair transplant surgery

Hair transplant surgery is an option, but is very expensive. It needs to be re-done as balding progresses, or you will be left with unsightly islands of restored hair in a sea of bare scalp.

If you are considering this procedure, always consult a properly qualified trichologist who is registered with the Institute of Trichologists (see www.trichologists.org.uk). Ensure that they are cosmetically and medically trained.

A trichologist can advise you on the nature of your balding, and the best treatment for it, including the best kind of hair transplant.

Next, you must choose a surgeon and discuss your expectations with them. A hair transplant, no matter how expensive, will only reduce bald patches using your own hair – it won't give you a new, thick head of hair.

Hair transplant surgery has improved massively in recent decades, thanks to the increasingly incremental way in which it can be done. The infamous "plug" grafts of the 1970s (which looked like strips of turf) have been replaced by mini and even micrografts, where hairs are inserted into incisions no bigger than a pinhole. Hair grafts work by harvesting not just a hair follicle, but a tiny part of the skin it grew from, and using it to replace a tiny part of skin where the follicle has died.

These grafts are usually harvested from the back of the patient's head, where the hair grows thickest and where they will hardly be missed.

The donor area, containing bald-resistant hairs, is trimmed before a section is selected for harvesting. This section, usually a wide, narrow strip of hair follicles, is then cut away and the incision sutured.

Hair is combed over the wound of the donor area, which is almost instantly invisible. Even when the hair is combed up, it will only appear as a thin, bald strip.

The cut-away tissue is then dissected into mini and micrografts. These are adhered via tiny incisions to the bald areas using an irregular pattern to appear more natural.

Typically, a surgeon uses micrografts to create a new hairline and minigrafts (comprising three to six hairs each) behind the hairline. You might need 250 or 3000 of these grafts, depending on the size of the area to be treated. This is why price can vary so much.

Following surgery, the patient will have a short, stubbly hair covering. The scalp will be red and might form scabs. Within a week, the redness and scabbing will mostly have disappeared and the hair will have started to grow.

Further transplants will have to be conducted to avoid patchiness as balding progresses.

Hair transplant surgery often costs between £3000 and £7000, depending on how extensive the area is and how many procedures are needed. (Some celebrities have been reported to have spent up to £30,000 on new hair!)

££ Salon and make-up counter

Minoxidil

Minoxidil is a popular product for reducing hair loss. It was originally formulated as a pharmaceutical treatment for high blood pressure, but it proved to have the interesting side-effect (in some cases) of slowing down or even reversing hair loss. No-one quite understands how it works, but formulations containing five per cent Minoxidil can be effective in treating small areas of male pattern baldness on men under 40.

According to surveys, it seems to work on approximately one third of those who have tried it. Some gain good regrowth, ohers experience a little regrowth of fine, wispy hair, while others experience no change.

Side-effects are mild and include rashes, headaches and palpitations, all of which can be treated.

Finasteride

Another popular product is Finasteride, This works by blocking the enzyme that causes the conversion of testosterone into DHT, so (in theory) no DHT equals no hair loss.

Finasteride is available on prescription only, and comes in tablet form. It must be used continuously to have a permanent effect. It takes from three to six months for improvement to become apparent, and improvement stops from six to 12 months after discontinuation of use.

Side-effects, though quite rare, are a bit more serious than with Minoxidil. These include a lowering of the sex drive, erectile dysfunction, breast tenderness and enlargement, rashes, testicular pain, and swelling of the lips and face. All of these side-effects disappear with discontinuation of product usage.

Anti-Androgens

Anti-androgens work by using hormonal drugs to block the action of DHT, and should only be used under medical supervision.

Anti-DHTs work by preventing the conversion of testosterone into DHT, and are widely available, usually as hair creams or lotions. Inhairit and Revivogen are two examples.

Anti-DHTs have mild or no side-effects.

Super oxide dismutase treatments

Super oxide dismutase treatments (or SODs for short) tackle super oxides. Super oxides are produced when the action of DHT triggers an immune response in the scalp. Super oxides treat hair follicles as foreign bodies and attack them.

In theory, using SODs to get rid of Super Oxides, prevents this attack on the follicles and therefore stops hair loss. In many cases, SODs also stimulate hair growth.

It is a topical treatment and comes in various forms, including Folligen and Tricomin.

£ Lifestyle and natural remedies

If your hair loss is down to male pattern baldness, then there is little you can do to prevent it or slow it down. It's all down to genes.

If there are other causes, there are things you can do.

Iron supplements

Anaemia is caused by a lack of iron in the diet. This is easily remedied by taking an iron supplement that your GP can prescribe for you.

Fungal infections

Fungal infections are easily treated with anti-fungal medicine. Ask your GP for advice.

Stress

Stress can be managed, and although self-help books may be useful, your GP might be the best source of guidance on this.

Side-effects

If hair loss is caused by the use of certain medications, consult your GP about possible alternatives.

Balanced diet

Meanwhile, overall good hair care, a balanced diet (containing plenty of protein, fresh fruit and vegetables) and regular, vigorous exercise will help to preserve your general good health and also keep your skin and scalp in good condition.

Hair products

There are also many hair products to help volumise thinning hair or techniques to lift hair at the roots, and a good hairdresser will advise you best.

Haircut

Finally, a clever haircut can do much to minimise the impact of baldness. Long, straggling locks combined with bald areas is a bad mix, magnifying the impact of the sparser areas.

Short, hair reduces the contrast with bald areas and looks neat and healthy.

Hair loss (women)

Female hair loss is much rarer than male hair loss, but no less devastating. It is generally experienced as an overall thinning, or as bald patches across the head, rather than the receding hairline and crown baldness typical of male pattern baldness.

Alopecia areata is hair loss caused by an auto-immune disease, triggering white blood cells to attack hair follicles. This causes hair growth to slow down and sometimes to stop altogether. It doesn't actually kill the follicles, which means that the hair can start to regrow in the future – which it often does.

There is no cure at present for alopecia areata, but it usually goes away without treatment.

Thinning of the hair can also result from hormones triggered by pregnancy, the menopause and severe dieting.

It is not immediately obvious, and the first sign is often extra hair in the hairbrush after brushing or in the plughole after hair-washing. Again, this may go away all by itself. This is particularly the case with post-pregnancy hair loss, which usually settles down and reverses within a year of the birth.

But not all female hair loss corrects itself naturally, and the prospect of baldness can severely cripple self-esteem and even lead to depression.

£££ Cosmetic procedures

Unfortunately, hair transplants are not generally suitable for women because they treat large, bald areas and women experience hair loss in patches or as a general thinning.

££ Salon and make-up counter

Minoxidil

Minoxidil is available in formulations especially for women, but the caveats apply to women too (see page 158). It can work, but not for everyone.

Finasteride

Finasteride is not recommended for women who are pregnant or are trying to become pregnant because it can damage an unborn child. A number of women have taken part in a clinical trial to test this product, and it has shown some success. However, these women had to take the contraceptive pill while on the trial to ensure they did not become pregnant. Finasteride remains unavailable to women to date because of the risks involved.

Volumising shampoos

Volumising shampoos and conditioners are highly recommended for post-pregnant and menopausal thinning because they can give hair added body and counteract some of the visual impact of hair loss.

Wigs and hairpieces

Six out of ten women who buy and wear wigs don't have hair loss at all, but simply wear them to achieve a different, high-glamour look. Go to a specialist wig-maker.

If hair loss is specific to certain areas, you can opt for custom-made hairpieces. Removable hairpieces are attached to surrounding hair or scalp using double-sided tape and can be taken off at night. Permanent pieces are attached used a specially formulated adhesive, and can withstand vigorous activity, showering and swimming.

£ Lifestyle and natural remedies

Healthy diet

Severe dieting and iron deficiency can sometimes contribute to hair loss in women, so a diet rich in iron – including liver and kidney, leafy green vegetables, soya products, fatty acids, protein and zinc – can make a huge difference. It can take many weeks to see a difference, so persevere.

Hair styling

Over-styling can weaken hair and lead to minor hair loss, so avoid bleaching and perms. Instead use natural hair dyes (including henna) which are available from high street chemists. Avoid blow-drying and over-vigorous brushing, and treat yourself to a scalp massage every other week to stimulate blood flow to the scalp.

Excess hair

See Facial Hair (page 116) for methods of removal of excess body hair.

£££ Cosmetic procedures

Laser treatment (page 116) and electrolysis (page 117) are effective.

££ Salon and make-up counter

Waxing (page 117) and sugaring (page 117), depilation creams (page 96), shaving (page 119), hair bleaching (page 118).

£ Lifestyle and natural remedies

There is little you can do through lifestyle changes to remove excess body hair.

Excess body hair and facial hair can be a symptom of Polycystic Ovary Syndrome (PCOS) in women. See your doctor if you have any suspicion that you might be suffering from this condition. Other symptoms include, excess weight, absence of or irregular periods, thinning hair on the head and acne.

The Body

A beautiful body has never been so easy to achieve, if you have the money, thanks to advances in cosmetic surgery. If you don't have the money the only sensible answer is to try to achieve a healthy, active lifestyle.

For those of you with busy family life and hectic work environment you'll know that "simply" changing your lifestyle can be one of the hardest things you'll ever try to do.

Theoretically all you need to do is eat a bit more fruit and take a bit more exercise to make improvements in your health. But for some people achieving a healthy lifestyle may require drastic reorganisation of time, changing job or having some "serious chats" at home. Why do you think the diet industry is such a lucrative business? There's no quick fix. Unless you can afford the surgery.

There are, however, achievable longterm lifestyle fixes that you will end up enjoying, even though they are hard to do initially, because they will make life better.

Excess fat

Carrying too much weight can destroy self-esteem and stores up all kinds of medical problems for the future – including coronary heart disease, Type II diabetes and some forms of cancer.

If you are overweight, you're not alone.

The World Health Organisation calculates that by 2015, 2.3 billion people will be overweight, and 700 million of them will be obese. The Body Mass Index (BMI) system is the most accurate means of establishing your ideal weight. To calculate your BMI, take your weight in kilograms and divide it by the square of your height in metres. If you score between 18 and 25, then your BMI is ideal. If you score above 25 you are overweight. If you score above 30 you are obese.

If you want to lose weight, you need to use more calories than you consume every day until the weight is lost. You can then maintain your target weight through a careful diet.

£££ Cosmetic procedures

Surgery is only suitable for those who are excessively overweight and are unable to lose it without some serious help. Bariatric surgery comes in two forms – gastric bypass and gastric banding. No form of surgery is without risk and being severely overweight adds to this risk.

Gastric bypass

Gastric bypass – also known as stomach stapling – works by reducing food intake and the amount of food you absorb. It is possible to lose up to two thirds of your bodyweight within two years using this procedure.

A gastric bypass operation takes between one and four hours and requires a general anaesthetic.

Both Roux-en-Y gastric bypass and biliopancreatic diversion bypass work by stapling the stomach to create a small pouch. This is then hooked up directly to the Y-shaped part of the small intestine, by-passing much of it to reduce food absorption. The small stomach pouch ensures that only small amounts of food can be ingested at any one time and that the food is well chewed.

However, weight loss is not automatic and you must adhere to a strict (often medically supervised) diet that includes supplementary vitamins. You will also have to commit to a specially devised exercise programme. If you continue to eat high-fat, high sugar food, then you probably won't lose any weight at all.

Recovery from a gastric bypass includes a few days in hospital, usually on a clear fluids diet. You will then have a recovery period of five weeks when your abdomen will probably feel very swollen and sore.

The procedure costs from £7500.

Gastric banding

Gastric banding is considerably less invasive because it

can be performed using keyhole surgery.

The procedure takes from 30 minutes to an hour. The surgeon makes several tiny incisions in the lower abdomen to insert the instruments that will put the band in place and create a small pouch at the upper end of the stomach.

This small pouch forces the patient to eat small meals and to chew their food well, or they will feel or actually be sick.

It is a permanent procedure. Again, it requires the application of a strict but healthy diet to really show results.

Gastric banding prices start at £5000.

Intragastric Balloon

The intragastric balloon is less invasive still. A balloon is inserted into the stomach and then filled with 400–700 cc of saline. Like gastric banding, it forces the patient to eat less.

This procedure costs around £4500.

Liposuction

If you only want to lose stubborn deposits of fat on areas like thighs, jowls, chin, upper arms, abdomen and hips, then liposuction is a popular option. (See pages 35 and 85.)

It will not make an obese person thin, but can make a formerly obese person feel good about their body.

Following a general anaesthetic, a stainless steel cannula

is inserted through a small incision at the problem site and fat is broken up and removed using a suction machine.

Tumescent liposuction is a variation on the tradition method. Here, fluid is injected into the fat, helping to separate it from the muscle and thus making it easier to remove. This also reduces the level of blood loss.

In Ultrasound-Assisted Liposuction (UAL) the cannula emits ultrasonic energy, which liquefies the fat and again makes it easier to remove.

Liposuction typically causes swelling and bruising so you are usually advised to wear pressure garments after surgery to reduce this and speed up skin retraction. The results are permanent, so if you regain weight you will only do so in areas that haven't been treated.

Side-effects can include nerve damage and infection.

Regular liposuction costs from £1500 per session. UAL liposuction Costs from about £3000 per session,

Lipodissolve

A fat-dissolving injection or lipodissolve is another option, though it's not quite clear how it works. It seems to emulsify fat, which is then absorbed by the lymphatic system and excreted.

The active ingredient in the injections is phosphatidylcholine (PC), which is derived from soya beans. Unlike liposuction, it doesn't permanently remove fat cells, so if you regain weight you will also regain it in the areas you had treated.

Visible improvement can take from one to four sessions, at around 45 minutes each.

Lipodissolve costs from £200 to £500 per session.

££ Salon and make-up counter

See products listed for cellulite on page 84.

£ Lifestyle and natural remedies

Losing weight gradually through healthy eating and exercise is the best, cheapest option. Some would say the only sensible option.

Get your head sorted

Successful losers change their lifestyle, they don't "go on a diet". People who "go on a diet" think they can "come off" the diet. "I'll start again on Monday." Forget that kind of thinking. You have to change the way you eat and the way you think about food **forever** or you'll be one of the many dieters who put back on all the weight they lose ... and more. (A 2007 study by UCLA found that, after 2 years, 85% of the dieters in their study had put the weight they'd lost back on – and 50% weighed even more.)

Don't kid yourself about having a slow metabolism. You are fat because you consume too many calories. You may think you don't eat that much, but **what** are you eating? Or, you might have a good healthy diet ... just far too much of a good healthy diet. Be totally honest about what you are eating and keep a food diary.

Weight loss surgery may successfully shift all the fat you've always hated but the reasons for the overeating might remain. You might not reach that elusive happy place you thought you were going to reach by getting thin, because being thin doesn't necessarily mean being happy, no matter what you might tell yourself.

If you feel your problem is emotional overeating, comfort eating or bingeing then you're going to need a bit of extra help. There are many support groups out there and your doctor may be able to help put you in touch with a counsellor, though NHS waiting lists can be long.

If there are stressful things in your life that make you feel the need to comfort yourself with food, they need to be sorted out first. You can't do two things at once, it's too hard. A few blips along the way are all part of the process – not a reason to give up. You are human not a robot.

Be kind to yourself – don't speak negatively to yourself. That little voice in your head that says: "You'll never do it", "you look hideous" needs to be banished forever. You wouldn't speak to your friends like that, so don't speak to yourself like that.

Support
If you feel you need help and support or some good natured nagging, you might want to try a slimming club. Organisations like Weightwatchers (www.weightwatchers.

co.uk), Slimming World (www.slimmingworld.com) and Scottish Slimmers (www.scottishslimmers.com), emphasise steady progress, a varied diet and good, healthy foodstuffs. They don't do gimmicks.

Dieting alongside others – online or at class – can give you much needed support during times when your weight reaches a plateau, or if you are making small, unwanted gains.

Eat healthily

Opt for small, regular meals, and never skip breakfast, which kickstarts your metabolism in the morning.

Eat plenty of fresh fruit and vegetables and high fibre foods (such as wholemeal bread, brown rice, wholewheat pasta, oats, beans and pulses). Avoid full-fat milk and butter and grill and poach instead of frying.

Get your five-a-day. In fact get more than five. Vegetables in general have so few calories in them that you can eat them freely (with the exception of potatoes and other starchy veg). Snack on fruit instead of biscuits.

Cut out refined flours, sugars and alcohol. Read up on the glycemic index and glycemic loading. Big variations in blood sugar are bad for you and can exacerbate cravings and mood swings.

Habit

Dr James Hill of the University of Colorado and Dr Rena Wing of the University of Pittsburgh set up the National

Weight Control Registry in 1993. It tracks about 3000 people who have lost at least 30 pounds and kept it off for a year or longer. They found, according to Dr Hill, that "to keep lost weight off, people must change their approach to exercise and develop new habits." They found the main habits of successful losers were:

- Eating a low-fat, high-carbohydrate diet
- Eating breakfast every day
- Monitoring weight regularly
- Keeping a food diary
- Getting about an hour of physical exercise every day, often just from walking
- And, crucially, they made this behaviour permanent.

Exercise

It's also important to exercise. Build up to a vigorous session of at least 30 minutes three times a week. Anything – but make sure you really enjoy it or you won't keep it up. Power walking is a great start and won't cost you more than a good pair of shoes. Even if it is not burning hundreds of calories, exercise is a mood lifter and will help alleviate the desire to comfort eat.

Choose life not food!

One last thing – **never** use being fat as an excuse for not doing what you want in life. Choose life, and being active and enjoyably busy helps ensure that food doesn't take on undue importance in your life.

Underdeveloped physique

Thinness and underdeveloped muscles can make even a fit body look puny and unhealthy. Many people – especially young men – think that an underdeveloped physique makes them undesirable and affects their confidence.

There are options available to help an underdeveloped physique.

£££ Cosmetic procedures

Pectoral implants

Pectoral implants is one of the most popular cosmetic procedures for men. Implants give better definition to existing chest muscles, and they can be a solution for those who simply cannot develop those muscles either because of their genetic make-up or because of injury.

The implants are solid silicone, which cannot rupture. (Silicone breast implants are fluid filled, and can rupture.)

Though the implants are solid, they have a certain degree of pliability and therefore feel like real muscle. They are available in a variety of shapes and sizes and can also be custom-made.

This procedure requires a general anaesthetic. The surgeon makes incisions in the armpits to minimise visible scarring. They then create a pocket underneath the existing pectoral muscles and insert the implant. Dissolving sutures hold the implant in place initially, and the resultant internal scar tissue takes over from there.

Surgery takes one to two hours. You should expect to feel discomfort and pain after the anaesthetic wears off, and to experience swelling and bruising for several more weeks.

Risks include the usual post-operative complications such as bleeding and infection and the accumulation of fluids around the implant. The application of drains immediately after the operation will prevent this.

These implants are permanent.

Pectoral implants cost around £7500.

Calf implants

Calf implants are an option for those who cannot develop their calf muscles, and feel that their legs look out of kilter with the rest of their body.

As with pectoral implants, the surgeon makes incisions and inserts the solid silicone implants in the creases behind the knees, into the pockets overlying the gastrocnemius muscle. This is a two-headed muscle, so two implants are usually inserted. However, if the patient has a condition such as bow-leggedness, then only one is required.

After surgery you need to keep your legs elevated for a two or three days to allow swelling to subside. You should also elevate your legs when you are resting for several days after this.

One side-effect is that the skin over the implant can

initially look shiny and stretched. This will gradually disappear, and the skin should end up looking quite natural.

The risks associated with this procedure are the same as for pectoral muscles.

Full recovery takes up to six weeks and the procedure is permanent

Calf implants cost around £2000.

Buttock implants

Buttock implants are available if you want a more defined buttock area, or if your buttocks are asymmetrical.

The incisions are made midway between the buttocks. The buttock muscle (or gluteus maximus) is then raised to allow the solid silicone implant to be inserted into a specially created pocket in the tissue.

Sutures hold the implant in place and bandages are usually applied for the short-term.

As you sit on your buttocks a lot of the time, post-operative recovery can be uncomfortable and requires a full six weeks. As the muscles stretch, the buttocks will look more natural, although this can take a few months. The procedure is permanent.

The risks associated with this procedure are the same as for pectoral muscles.

Buttock implants cost from £5000.

££ Salon and make-up counter

There are no beauty products available for an underdeveloped physique.

£ Lifestyle and natural remedies

Developing muscle is not as daunting as it might seem. Needless to say, you should never use anabolic steroids to do it.

Gym

The first step is to find a good gym and a reputable trainer. If you plan to follow a regime of targeted exercise you need to learn to do the exercises well and understand how to build on your progress.

You might only need to employ a personal trainer on an occasional basis. That way, you can keep your costs down.

Exercises such as bench presses, flys using weights, push-ups, machine dips and machine pullovers are recommended for pectoral muscles.

Calf raises are the best way to develop your calf muscles. However, these exercises are hard-going, painful and require serious persistence because your calf muscles are the most difficult to develop.

Be aware that muscles grow while resting, not training, so exercising every day will not get you the results you want – rather, the reverse, because overworked muscle fibre simply breaks down. So either work different muscles on different days, or do a full work-out on alternate days.

A good diet is also essential. Don't bother with so-called muscle drinks. Instead, eat a varied and balanced diet with the emphasis on lean protein (for example white fish) and iron (for example, green leafy vegetables).

Eat plenty of wholegrains and fresh produce and keep yourself well-hydrated and well-rested.

Eat little and often rather than having big meals three times a day, and avoid fat and sugar as much as you can. Sports drinks are recommended during exercise as their typical combination of carbohydrates and protein helps to reduce muscle damage.

Breast augmentation

Many women feel that their breasts are either underdeveloped, or that they have lost volume following pregnancy and breastfeeding. As a result, they feel less feminine and less sexually attractive. This can lead them to feel so painfully self-conscious that they avoid wearing revealing clothing or swimwear.

A mastectomy can leave a woman feeling bereft, as the loss of a breast can feel like the loss of part of her identity. Asymmetry is another reason why women may seek breast augmentation of some kind.

The most obvious and popular solution is surgical enhancement. As with any surgical procedure, take care to choose a reputable surgeon and never make your decision based on cost.

There are also other remedies apart from surgery for small and sagging breasts.

£££ Cosmetic procedures

First of all, you should think carefully about what size you hope to achieve, and take advice on this. Ideally, wear padding up to the desired size to see how it looks in proportion to the rest of your body and don't trust a surgeon who agrees with you that a double DD cup size will look fine on a size 8 body. If you have small breasts, then even one cup size up will make a big difference.

Breast implants

Look for a good surgeon with plenty of reliable testimonials, and be careful when choosing the size and shape of your implants and the material they are made of.

Saline implants remain popular. They are filled with sterile saltwater, which will be harmlessly reabsorbed by the body if they rupture. The other advantage is that they can be filled on-site, so precise individual requirements can be met.

Silicone implants are soft and fluid, but are pre-filled. Cohesive gel implants are a newer kind of implant. These are more stable than saline implants – if they rupture, the gel will retain its shape. They also have the advantage of giving a more natural, softer feel and look.

All implants come with a silicone rubber outer shell, known as a lumen.

Surgery is conducted under general anaesthetic and takes one to two hours. Incisions are usually made beneath the breast, though they can be made in the armpit or around the nipple area.

Implants are then placed either in a pocket created behind the breast tissue, or in one created behind the pectoral muscle, next to the chest wall. When treating asymmetry probably only one implant is required.

The incisions are then sutured and taped to keep them in place, and the breasts wrapped in gauze or a surgical bra. Swelling and bruising lasts a few days. Full recovery takes around two weeks.

Scarring can take up to two years to fade fully, though redness should subside within six weeks.

Risks – other than the usual post-operative complications – include rupturing, which causes the breast to suddenly look deflated. This can only be corrected by a further surgical procedure.

The presence of breast implants can hinder the early detection of breast cancer. Be aware of this, and ensure that you have regular mammograms and that your radiographer is familiar with implants and the need to X-ray them carefully.

Finally, a rare side-effect of breast implants is temporary or even permanent loss of sensation.

Implants are not permanent. Breast tissue will start to sag over the years, so you might need another breast-lift in the future.

Costs range from £4000 to £7000.

££ Salon and make-up counter

Pills

Health shops and websites sell herbal supplements and pills that claim to increase your cup size.

Herbal pills claim to work by using plant extracts to mimic oestrogen. Oestrogen stimulates the growth of breast tissue at puberty and during pregnancy.

The ingredients of these pills include fenugreek (used to boost the milk supply of nursing mothers), saw palmetto berry (used to boost breast tissue growth and relieve PMS), black cohosh root extract, dong quai root, blessed thistle, dandelion root, watercress leaf, fennel seed and kelp.

If you respond to these ingredients, then you will see results within four to eight weeks, and maximum improvement within six months.

Breast creams

Breast creams claim to work in much the same way by stimulating breast tissue growth. The active ingredients are similar to herbal pills. Being topical, they may be safer, and generally require daily application, for several months or more.

None of these products are suitable for pubescent girls or women who are pregnant or breastfeeding.

£ Lifestyle and natural remedies

Exercise

As the breasts are comprised entirely of fat cells, milk ducts and glands no amount of targeted exercise will actually make them any bigger. But you can make them look bigger, by strengthening the muscles that support them.

Use the same exercises as recommended for pectoral muscles (page 183). Please note that women who are not seeking to bulk up muscle should use hand-held weights no heavier than 3 to 5 lbs.

Bra

Your choice of bra can also make a huge difference. A properly fitted bra with the correct size cup can have a miraculous effect. If your weight is fluctuating be sure to get measured regularly, and it makes sense to ask advice if it is available (most good department stores and lingerie shops will have an expert on hand to measure you and make recommendations as to size and style).

Padded bras are very sophisticated and ideal for those who want a bit of boost when they are wearing a low-cut top. Water or gel-filled bras give a natural feel and look and are remarkably comfortable. A department store with a good lingerie department should meet all your needs.

Breast reduction (women)

Breasts that are too large can cause pain in the back, shoulders and neck. If they are left as they are, they can cause serious muscular problems in later life.

Breasts that are considered much larger than normal can cause enormous mental and physical discomfort. Properly fitting bras and clothes can be almost impossible to come by, bra-straps can leave deep, red grooves in the shoulders and lack of confidence can lead to debilitating depression. In addition, heavy folds of breast tissue against the skin of the torso can cause excessive sweating and soreness, and can allow fungal infections to thrive.

Sports and other physical activities are greatly hindered, as is early detection of breast cancer.

For all these reasons, breast reduction operations are often available on the NHS and if these issues affect you, speak to a sympathetic GP first, rather than a cosmetic surgeon.

£££ Cosmetic procedures

Breast reduction surgery

Breast reduction surgery (or reduction mammoplasty) should begin with an extensive consultation, during which you can discuss the ideal size and shape of your post-op breasts and the risks and benefits of surgery.

Surgery begins with the administration of a general

anaesthetic. An initial incision is made around the nipple area, a second incision is made on a vertical down to the crease beneath the breast, and a third along this crease, creating an anchor-shaped incision pattern. If the breasts are very large, the nipple may be removed entirely and then re-attached in what is known as a free nipple graft. Usually, however, the nipple remains attached to the deep breast tissue as it is re-positioned.

The areola might be trimmed at this stage if the surgeon thinks that they are overly large. The next step is to remove excess breast tissue, either through sharp dissection or liposuction. The skin will also be trimmed, if necessary.

Sutures are then made in a deeply layered pattern through the breast tissue. This provides support while healing.

The procedure takes from two to four hours. Scarring is initially very visible and your surgeon should prepare you for this. It should fade completely after two years.

Swelling and bruising last for up to two weeks. After this, you should be able to see the size and shape of your new breasts.

Reduction mammoplasty carries some risks. These include scarring, temporary or permanent loss of sensation and asymmetry (including nipples not being level). Many women are unable to breastfeed following breast reduction surgery, so discuss this with your surgeon if you plan to start a family.

Further risks include partial or even total loss of the nipple and areola, skin discolouration or changes in pigment and damage to underlying muscle and tissue.

If you gain weight or become pregnant after surgery, this will also affect the results.

Many women are very satisfied with the results of reduction mammoplasty, and can face life with vastly increased confidence and physical comfort.

As with breast implants, the price range starts at £4000, moving up into the region of £7000. Many breast reduction operations are done following an NHS referral.

££ Salon and make-up counter

There are no beauty products available that can reduce the size of breasts.

£ Lifestyle and natural remedies

Lose weight

See pages 176–179 for advice on weight loss. Big breasts can be the result of carrying too much weight in general, so it's essential to achieve a healthy Body Mass Index. If your breasts are still disproportionately large and you find this difficult to live with, then surgery might be your only recourse.

Breast reduction (men)

Over recent years, there has been an increase in the number of men seeking breast reduction surgery for gynaecomastia. Male breast development, or "man boobs" as they are crudely known, should not be confused with excessive fatty tissue caused by obesity. Gynaecomastia is a condition characterised by a man's development of glandular breast tissue – similar to that of a woman's – resulting in the formation of smallish breasts.

Environmental factors (such as the increasing use of oestrogen as a growth hormone in the meat industry, and the excretion of oestrogen by female users of the contraceptive pill into the water supply) could be to blame, though heredity may also play a part.

Other causes include hormonal changes (most boys experience some female-type breast development during puberty, though this usually subsides within a year), the use of hormone drugs, excessive alcohol consumption and severe starvation.

However, an overdeveloped breast or breasts can indicate an underlying medical cause so if this is the case, consult your GP before approaching a cosmetic surgeon.

Understandably, breast development in men – particularly young men – is extremely embarrassing and can cause self-consciousness and depression.

The good news is, you can do something about it.

£££ Cosmetic procedures

Liposuction

If it is just a case of excess fatty deposits – pseudo-gynaecomastia – liposuction can be performed (see pages 35, 85 and 174). This should only be done when the patient has achieved a healthy weight, which he can maintain.

Liposuction only involves a minor incision to insert the cannula.

Surgery

The procedure is more extensive if there is glandular tissue, and begins with the administration of a general anaesthetic. An initial incision is made around the nipple area, and the nipple itself can be trimmed to make it look more masculine.

A second incision is then made in a wider, eye-shape around the nipple area, so that excess skin and tissue can be removed.

The incisions are then sutured. You'll probably be advised to wear a pressure garment post-op to lend support and aid skin retraction. Scarring is inevitable, but should be minimal because the incisions have followed the chest's natural contours.

Swelling and bruising should subside within a few days. Avoid vigorous activity for six weeks. Results will be fully apparent after three months.

Risks are rare, but are the same as those associated

with female breast reduction – the loss of the nipple, temporary or permanent loss of sensation and asymmetry. Darker skins may be at greater risk of keloid scarring (page 60).

Most patients are very satisfied with the results of their surgery and report a much improved quality of life thereafter.

Costs range from £3000 to £5000.

££ Salon and make-up counter

There are no beauty products available that will reduce breast size in men.

£ Lifestyle and natural remedies

Weight control

If you are overweight then you are more likely to develop breasts. Try to achieve the ideal weight for your height. See page 176 for advice on weight loss.

Side-effects

If weight is not an issue but you are taking medication, then ask your doctor about possible side-effects of a number of medications, including their potential to cause the development of female-like breasts. If you change or stop your medication, perhaps you could stop the problem.

Saggy breasts

Gravity, significant weight loss and pregnancy can result in breasts looking saggy, pendulous and ill-defined, with downward-pointing nipples.

£££ Cosmetic procedures

Mastopexy (or breastlift)

A mastopexy (or breastlift) differs from a breast augmentation in that it is concerned with the shape of the breasts, rather than the size. However, a breastlift can be done in conjunction with breast implants following (for example) pregnancy and breastfeeding, when breasts have lost shape, tone and volume.

The aim of the breastlift is to give you firmer, younger-looking breasts. As the name implies, it is a procedure that lifts and re-shapes, and can even include a re-positioning of the nipples and a trimming of the areola. It is most effective on small breasts because the less tissue you have to lift, the easier it is to do.

The procedure begins with a general anaesthetic. The surgeon then makes the same anchor-shaped incision pattern as for the breast reduction procedure. The nipple is raised while remaining attached to deeper breast tissue. The tissue is then re-shaped and excess skin removed.

At this stage, the areola area can also be trimmed.

Incisions are then closed and sutured in a layered pattern, as with the breast reduction procedure.

A breastlift takes between one and three hours to complete.

Scarring can be significant, but should fade rapidly. It should have disappeared by two years. If redness remains or scar tissue is obvious then this is probably due to your skin type rather than to the skill of the surgeon. Both can be hidden in even quite revealing swimwear.

Swelling and bruising last for a few days and you will probably be advised to wear a supportive or surgical bra. The results should be visible within a couple of weeks, with tenderness and pain subsiding within this time.

The risks are the same as for breast augmentation (see page 185), breast reductions (see page 190) and breast implants (see pages 186).

The results are not permanent and ageing may still cause the breasts to sag in future. You may be advised to wait until after having children before undertaking this procedure. Minimise future sagging by wearing good supportive underwear.

A breastlift costs from £4000, though this does not include the cost of implants.

££ Salon and make-up counter

Bust-firming creams

Bust-firming creams are widely available. These treat the

area from the crease beneath the breast right up to the chin – the so-called "natural bra".

The décolletage – the area including the cleavage upwards – is notoriously neglected in most skincare routines and is often where you see sun damage and age spots.

Furthermore, it is often pulled and stretched by pregnancy and the downward force of gravity.

Any intense moisturiser will help, but there are also dedicated creams available to try. Ingredients can include wheatgerm oil (for moisturising), radish (for toning) soya and jojoba and avocado oils (for nourishing) co-enzyme Q10 (for accelerating cell turnover) glycerin (for hydrating) and green tea (for anti-oxidant properties)

A bust firming cream is not plastic surgery in a jar, but at least it will improve skin tone in the area from your breasts to your chin.

Make-up

If all you are wanting is a lift for a special occasion, take some tips from the make-up artists. First, exfoliate the "natural bra" area gently, then moisturise and apply your facial foundation – ideally a matt formula. Take a bronzer (the same one you use for your cheekbones) and apply in the shadow of your cleavage, taking care to blend it in. Add – a dab of highlighter to the "moons" of the breasts as a finishing touch.

£ Lifestyle and natural remedies

Massage

Massage improves circulation and lymphatic drainage and keeps the skin looking healthy and toned. It must be done daily to make a difference, but this has the added bonus of familiarising you with your breast shape and idiosyncrasies and you will therefore be much more likely to spot lumps as soon as they appear.

Here are some techniques to try:

- Place one palm on either side of the nipple, then press both palms together against the flesh of the breast. Release. Repeat five times each side.
- Knead the breast gently, working round the nipple to complete a circle. Try this three times.
- Using fingers, smooth away from the nipple in a series of strokes till a circle has been completed. Again, repeat three times.

Exercise

Exercise can't alter breast tissue but exercising the surrounding muscles can improve the way your bust looks. Have a look at the exercises recommended for pectoral muscles (see page 183).

Bra

A good, supportive bra can help to stop breasts from sagging. It's particularly important to wear a well-fitted

Saggy breasts

maternity bra while pregnant and a well-fitted nursing bra while breastfeeding. Always get properly measured up after any major bodily change such as weight loss or childbirth, and never attempt even gentle sports without wearing a sports bra.

Droopy thighs

Over time, the skin of the thighs invariably becomes less toned, saggy and dimpled with cellulite. Age, gravity and genes are mainly to blame, though excessive UV exposure will reduce the skin's natural elasticity and neglect will compound the problem.

Rigorous diet and exercise regimes are long-term solutions. A thighlift is the short-cut, though it is not pain-free.

£££ Cosmetic procedures

Thighlift

To evaluate whether you are a good candidate for a thighlift, pull up the skin of your thigh. If there is a dramatic difference for the better, then it could be suitable for you. Thighlifts give thighs a leaner, smoother look, improve skin tone and general contour and are often done in combination with a buttock lift and abdominoplasty.

The fronts and sides of the thighs are very treatable with surgery, but the backs are less so.

The procedure begins with the administration of a general anaesthetic. The surgeon then makes a small incision in the groin area. (If you are having a minor thighlift on an outpatient basis this incision will be enough, but if you require a more major operation, this initial incision will extend downwards around the thigh.)

Scars are usually discreet, hidden by natural creases or the lines of lingerie and swimwear.

To tackle the outer thigh, a second incision is made, beginning in the groin area and extending outwards to the hip, in a line similar to that of a high-cut swimsuit.

The skin is then separated from the fat, and the fat from muscle. Excess fat is removed – either by being excised or by using liposuction – and the skin is pulled upwards and the excess trimmed. Incisions are sutured into place, including the underlying tissue to support the new contours created by the surgeon. Drains can be attached temporarily to remove excess fluid and a compression garment or bodystocking will probably be recommended to reduce swelling and aid skin retraction.

Thighlifts take between one and three hours. A minor lift requires only prescription painkillers and rest at home, while a major lift requires several days of hospital care, including painkilling injections and catheters. Bruising and swelling remain for up to a month. A full recovery takes from four to six months, though a return to work and even vigorous activity is possible within six weeks or so if there are no complications.

Risks include nerve damage, skin pigmentation and infection.

Most patients report a smoother, more youthful shape, although a healthy diet and a regular exercise regime are essential to maintain this.

Costs range from £4000 to £5500.

££ Salon and make-up counter

Creams

Thigh creams are available but there is no clear evidence to prove that they are effective. For example, Aminophylline, was formerly a drug prescribed to treat bronchial asthma. Recent claims are that its fat-dissolving properties can slim thighs. Commercial studies have so far been inconclusive. It can cause a nasty allergic reaction.

Caffeine

Caffeine is claimed to be a fat-buster. What it actually does is flush out cells, so the leaner look that results is caused by temporary dehydration. For treatment of dimpled skin, see the Cellulite section, page 84.

£ Lifestyle and natural remedies

Exercise

Exercise is essential to maintain toned thighs. Examples are walking, skipping with a skipping rope (ten minutes, three times a week) and a vigorous aerobics workout, which includes thigh-targeted exercises.

Yoga

Yoga is also recommended, as regular practice results in a leaner, longer shape.

Droopy upper arms

Droopy upper arms – also known as "bingo wings" and "bat wings" – are one of the body's first signs of ageing.

This problem is caused by age and gravity but fluctuating weight due to yo-yo dieting or pregnancies is also a contributory factor. Smoking, poor diet and a sedentary lifestyle makes matters worse.

Diet and exercise can help when the problem is just beginning, but once the bat wing is there it's hard to shift, because it is loose tissue rather than fat or muscle.

Surgery is one solution, but that isn't problem free.

£££ Cosmetic procedures

Brachioplasty (or upper arm lift)

A brachioplasty (or upper arm lift) will result in hundreds of sutures and extensive scarring that might not completely fade, since body skin tends to scar more severely than facial skin.

Surgery begins with either a local or general anaesthetic depending on whether you have chosen a major or minor upper arm lift.

The surgeon usually makes a curved or zigzagged incision from armpit to elbow in the inner surface of the upper arm.

The incision can also be made towards the back of the upper arm. This results in a longer scar that is less immediately visible. If it is a minor lift, then a smile-shaped incision in the armpit will probably suffice.

If excess fat deposits are an issue, then unwanted fatty tissue will be removed at this stage through excision or liposuction. Underlying tissue will then be sutured into place to create a new contour and to support skin.

The skin is then stretched and trimmed. The shape of the skin excision is usually triangular. Finally, the incision is sutured and taped to provide a little extra support.

Surgery takes one to three hours.

You will probably feel tightness in the arm area immediately after the operation, and will be advised to wear a support bandage to reduce swelling and aid skin retraction.

Sutures are removed within one to three weeks. Swelling and bruising subside within two to three weeks and a full recovery takes up to four months.

Risks include the usual post-operative complications including excessive bleeding, numbness and infection.

Added hazards include skin necrosis (i.e. when the tissue dies) along the scar. If necrosis should occur, the dead tissue would have to be surgically removed in a follow-up, corrective operation, and replaced with skin grafts.

Irregular contours may also result, as a result of necrosis or excessive tissue removal. Again, corrective surgery may be necessary.

Despite the risk of scarring, upper arm surgery is

usually successful and can result in a transformed appearance to the upper body.

Brachioplasty costs from £2000.

££ Salon and make-up counter

Creams

There are some upper arm firming creams available. These products usually work by forming a layer over the skin that shrinks as it dries, creating an instant toning effect.

Ingredients include sweet almond extract (said to have a lifting effect on saggy skin), fish oil (helps to promote healthy skin), elastin peptides (said to stimulate collagen production, giving skin greater resilience) and grapeleaf and blackcurrant (said to have firming properties).

Exfoliate your upper arms with a gentle body scrub using circular movements – this will boost circulation and should be done before applying the firming cream.

Although firming creams can make skin feel firmer and fresher, they cannot significantly reduce the appearance of loose skin – especially not the flaps that can develop under the triceps.

Fake tan and bronzer

Fake tan can help to slim upper arms, but you should apply it with care. Exfoliate first to smooth out bumps and spots then apply evenly with an application mitt.

If you haven't got a mit, wash your hands thoroughly – and quickly!

Another cosmetic trick is to apply bronzer to the flabby underside, creating a "shadow" and making arms appear leaner. Avoid short sleeves. Longer sleeves with flared cuffs can extend arms and deflect attention from the upper area.

£ Lifestyle and natural remedies

Exercise

Vigorous, regular exercise will keep you trim overall and help to prevent droopy underarms.

Rowing – or working out on the rowing machine at the gym – are especially effective.

Yoga is also ideal, as it makes your muscles longer and leaner and gives a better profile to legs and arms (including upper arms). Or stretch fully, raising your arms up above your head and hold at full extent for 20–30 seconds. Try this several times a day.

Press-ups and flys (with small weights) and flamenco dancing (with its emphatic arm movements) are also good for toning upper arm muscles.

Hands

We use them all the time, they're nearly always visible, yet we neglect them and, while your face may be youthful, your body trim and lithe and your hair bountiful, your lined and veiny hands will give the game away.

Hand care is the poor relation of facial skincare, and all too often, it shows. Because of exposure to sunlight, usually without sunscreen, hands are often the first place we witness age or liver spot formation, and as we age, and tissue thins, our hands can develop an elderly, bony cast long before the rest of us.

£££ Cosmetic procedures

Encourage new cell growth

The options for hand rejuvenation include chemical peels, which can help to reduce the appearance of age spots and encourage the growth of new, healthier-looking skin cells, by sloughing away the old ones.

Microdermabrasion will buff up skin, by removing the very fine outer layers, resulting in a fresher, more youthful appearance.

Laser skin resurfacing reduces age spots and also broken veins and other blemishes.

If you want to plump your hands up a little then one option is injectable fillers that include your own body fat or collagen.

Chemical peels and microdermabrasion prices start at around £60.

Laser treatment costs from £500 to £1000.

££ Salon and make-up counter

Exfoliate

The skin of the hands, like that of the face, should be exfoliated regularly to help cell turnover and keep skin looking fresh and clean. Products containing alpha-hydroxy acids (AHAs) work well, but they increase sun sensitivity. A simple body scrub or body soap is also effective, and should be used twice a week.

Moisturise

A nourishing hand cream is essential. You should apply it daily, or after handwashing, dishwashing or exposure to harsh winter weather.

Look out for intensely moisturising ingredients such as hemp oil, avocado oil, olive oil, coconut oil and shea butter.

For a moisturising boost, apply a generous amount of good quality hand cream last thing, before putting on cotton gloves. A number of good quality creams actually include a pair of gloves in the package. Overnight, your hands will receive a hydrating treatment that will keep them fresher-looking for days.

Skin lightening

Ingredients such as kojic acid can help to lighten age spots, as can daisy flower extract, which has brightening properties. Retinol is also an effective skin lightener, but as it also thins skin it should be used with caution because the skin on the hands tends to thin with age as it is.

£ Lifestyle and natural remedies

Protect your hands

If you wear gloves in cold weather you will not only keep your hands warm, but protect them, too,

Use rubber gloves when washing dishes or doing other household chores, because detergents and chemicals can leave skin red and itchy and seriously dehydrated.

Try zinc oxide, which is light and absorbent and serves as an effective barrier against weather and pollution.

Sunblock is also recommended – UV rays will damage skin no matter what you put on it at bedtime.

Feet

Wear high heels too often, and your feet can become seriously bashed out of shape and unfit to be seen.

General neglect can also leave feet looking less than their best, with cracked skin at the heels, ingrown toenails, and rough, hardened skin along the footbase.

However, it takes only minimal, regular care to transform less-than-perfect feet.

£££ Cosmetic procedures

Feet "nips and tucks" is a controversial new area in plastic surgery rejected by reputable cosmetic surgeons.

Surgeons have been asked to perform "toe tucks", to reduce the size of toes or to create a "cascade effect", where the toes reduce in size towards the pinkie in perfect gradations.

Then, there are the requests for surgery to heighten arches, for collagen or Botox injections in the footpad to numb the pain of wearing high heels, not to mention liposuction for slimmer ankles.

None of the above can ever be recommended.

And as for Botox and collagen – just remember that pain is one of the only ways your body can tell you that something is wrong, so shut it off at your peril.

££ Salon and make-up counter

Moisturise

A good foot moisturiser should include something like mint, or tea tree oil, both of which have cooling, disinfectant properties. Ingredients such as cocoa or shea butter will ensure that they are well moisturised.

For added benefit, put on a pair of socks immediately after application. Cream to treat cracked heels is widely available, but this is basically an effective moisturiser. Vaseline can be very effective too.

To soften up rough skin, invest in a good foot file and use it on clean, dry feet. Then moisturise your feet and wash the foot file using warm, soapy water, allowing it to air-dry thoroughly before putting away.

Exfoliate

Foot exfoliators are also effective, and should contain a good abrasive agent, such as pumice. Your feet can take it.

Foot soaks can be relaxing and those containing mint or tea tree oil will refresh your feet and help to stimulate the circulation.

£ Lifestyle and natural remedies

Choose shoes wisely

Save heels for special occasions, as nothing will disfigure

your feet faster. Shoes should be comfortable, with a thick sole to cushion your body against bumps and hard surfaces and a flexible upper, to allow your feet to bend as you walk.

Ensure your arches are supported. The sole of a shoe should be flexible but the arch should be firm. Where your feet bend your shoe can bend – where they do not your shoe should be firm and give proper support.

Hygiene

Change socks and tights every day, and keep feet scrupulously clean and dry, especially between the toes, where fungal infections can thrive. A regular six-monthly visit to a podiatrist is also recommended to prevent hard skin and ingrown toenails and to nip fungal and other infections in the bud.

Watch your weight

Obesity and insufficiently supportive shoes can lead to a condition of the foot called plantar fasciitis (inflammation of the muscle that runs along the sole of your foot). It is easier to try to avoid ever getting this condition than it is to try and treat it once you start to suffering from it. A regime of regular stretches and resting the feet is often the only cure and this can take months.

Carrying too much weight can cause the skin on the heels to harden and crack. Keep heels moisturised and exfoliated and try to keep your weight down (see page 176–179).

Fingernails

Your fingernails don't need to be long, blood-red talons to be beautiful. Trim, pink nails with clean, white tips look healthy and youthful. Bad nails – whether through habitual biting, infection or neglect – can detract from the most glamorous person's appearance.

£££ Cosmetic procedures

You don't need surgery to improve the look of your nails. If you have a nail disorder such as a fungal infection go to your GP as soon as possible as these types of disorders don't get better without medical treatment.

££ Salon and make-up counter

Salon treatments

Manicures are the most obvious salon treatment for nails, though you can learn to do it at home.

A nail technician will clean, file and shape your nails, soften up and shape cuticles, and finally buff nails to make them shine, and perhaps even paint on a coat of conditioning nail polish.

A manicure costs around £20, and should be repeated every month or so.

Artificial nails are a very popular cosmetic treatment, but they can damage your real nails.

Acrylic is the most popular material because it is hard-wearing yet malleable. Dedicated nail salons or good hair and beauty salons will be able to apply acrylics properly. Ask around before committing yourself.

An application session takes around half an hour and begins with the surface of the real nail being filed to create a rough surface. This makes it more receptive to the adhesive that will hold your acrylic nail in place. The new nail is then filed into shape and buffed to a good shine. The result is quite spectacular, giving you instant long, hard nails.

Nail care thereafter is fairly basic – apply a little oil from time to time to prevent brittleness and have new acrylics applied every six weeks or so before new, natural nail growth becomes too obvious.

Acrylic nail kits

Acrylic nail kits mean that you can do the work at home, but buy quality ones and always apply to scrupulously clean nails.

Nail thickeners

Weak nails – characterised by peeling, splitting and flaking – can be treated with nail thickeners (sometimes billed as nail hardeners or strengtheners). Good ingredients include retinol, wheat protein and calcium.

Cuticle remover

Damaged cuticles can spoil the appearance of nails. Choose a cuticle remover or softener containing sweet almond oil and nourishing vitamins A and E. Cuticle remover softens the problem skin and enables you to push it back with an orange stick without damaging it.

Damaged cuticles can be painful, can harm nails and even hinder growth, so treat them gently.

Nail whitener

If nails are yellow, either naturally or because of overuse of nail polish, for example, then a nail whitener can help. This is a soaking solution, and should include a brightening agent such as licorice.

£ Lifestyle and natural remedies

Diet

Bad nails are often attributable to bad dietary habits, so cut down on alcohol and cigarettes, and take in plenty of zinc, calcium and iron.

Stop biting!

If you bite your nails you should try to stop. Nail biting can damage nails in the long term and lead to nasty infections. Formulae to prevent nail biting are usually bitter-tasting but harmless substances.

Protect

Rubber gloves are a must when doing housework or cleaning, as these will protect nails from the damaging effects of household detergents.

Hygiene

Keep nails clean using a good, soft nailbrush and a mild soap. To push back cuticles, soak nails in warm water and use nothing harder than your own (clean) nail to press them back.

Trim your nails or, better still, file them into shape, trimming off rag nails to prevent infection.

Hand cream will keep hands soft and nourish nails too. Look for hand creams with built-in nail conditioner.

The End?

There are some things that are universally good for most of the complaints and worries we have about ourselves. Some have been touched on briefly in the different sections of this book. Let's visit them before we end this book.

Confidence

We've looked at lots of things we can do to physically improve how we look. One sure way to look better, that we haven't touched on too much, one that is probably more important than all the rest, is this: improving how you feel. A happy, confident, kind person will glow more radiantly than the most empirically beautiful model.

Lack of self confidence can feel overwhelming. It is beyond the scope of this book to list the strategies you can use to improve confidence but, be assured, there are plenty. Another volume in this series, *Positive Thinking, Positive Living* by Dr David Fong, has all the advice you need to start thinking in a new way.

Confidence, assertiveness and positivity can be learned. Your GP can help, but there are also hundreds of books available on the subject. Look at www.mind.org.uk and www.mentalhealth.org.uk for guidance.

Sleep

One of the best gifts you can give your body is to get a decent sleep. Many of us find sleeping for that magic eight hours a night to be near impossible – whether because we can't resist watching TV till the early hours, or because we feel we have to work long into the night to meet deadlines, or because we can't switch off because of stress. Sometimes there's no obvious reason for the insomnia. There are theories that lack of sleep can cause or exacerbate various health problems: obesity, diabetes, heart problems and depression being some of them.

In addition it hampers your ability to pay attention and learn new things. It increases your risk of making mistakes and you risk falling asleep at the wheel of your car while driving.

Again, there are whole books dedicated to strategies for beating the often debilitating disorder of insomnia, but below we have a few tips here to help get the most from the hours where we are *meant* to be sleeping.

Wind down for an hour before bedtime. Set an alarm an hour before bed. Prepare for bedtime like it's a major event of the day – which it is, really. At seven to eight hours duration, sleeping is a third of your day.

Before bed, get your things ready for the next day. Let this become part of a routine of simplifying the morning and introducing calm to your day.

The natural Circadian rhythm of the body is important and it is because of this that experts advise an hour of sleep before midnight is worth two after.

Sleep is something free to us all, and several weeks of eight hours a night, will help most of us.

If you are exercising more and have begun a new regime, bear in mind your body will need more rest.

A hot milky drink, or herbal tea with camomile can

aid getting into a sleepy or meditative state. Make sure your bedroom is well ventilated and low lit. Turn off all electronic devices. If you are going through a stressful time, extra sleep can help you recover and prepare for the following day.

See sleepfoundation.org and www.mentalhealth.org.uk for good advice on sleep and sleep disorders.

Hydration, nutrition and activity

Water is essential for our existence. Staying hydrated is cheap and easy and good for the skin (if you don't want wrinkles, drink water). Water from the tap is free and safe in the UK, and more eco-friendly than buying plastic bottles of mineral water. About 8–10 glasses a day is about right, no need for more.

Another 'simple' thing you can do for yourself is eat healthily and keep active (see pages 176–179). Make a point of moving every day – a 30-minute walk will do. Eat plenty of fruit and vegetables, choose low GI carbohydrates, eat palm-sized portions of protein and stay away from processed ready-meals, refined carbs, glucose, trans fats and junk food. Easy! With our busy lifestyles it is of course never really that easy to do the right thing all the time. But changing a bad diet into a good one can make a huge difference to mind and body.

There's no space here to give you a detailed eating and exercise plan, however why not look at www.nhs.uk/Livewell/healthy-eating and www.nhs.uk/livewell/fitness for good sensible advice.

INDEX

223